Praise for
Amy B. Scher's Previous Books

This Is How I Save My Life

"Amy Scher is a brave warrior and a wonderful writer. She is a living example (very much living!) of what it looks like when a woman takes her health, her heart, and her destiny into her own hands. My hope is that this book will inspire many other women to do the same."

Elizabeth Gilbert
#1 *New York Times* bestselling author
of *Eat Pray Love* and *Big Magic*

"A heartwarming and inspiring story that will change the way you look at life."

Vikas Swarup
New York Times bestselling author
of *Slumdog Millionaire*

"Amy Scher goes to the edge of losing herself in mind, body, and spirit, and shows us that . . . sometimes it takes traveling to the other side of the globe to discover what was right in front of us all along."

Laura Munson
New York Times bestselling author of
This Is Not the Story You Think It Is . . .

"A homecoming of healing, a human story of finding faith, wrapped in a blanket of humor and page-turning candor."

Kristen Noel
editor-in-chief of Best Self

"This is the rare book that is both breezy and deep. It speaks to the magic of international travel and how it can tempt and taunt you to expand into the very best version of yourself, or perhaps become someone entirely new."

Adam Skolnick
author of *One Breath* and over thirty
Lonely Planet travel guides

"In her stunning new memoir, *This Is How I Save My Life*, the refrain 'we are the healing we've been waiting for' rings throughout . . . A beautiful testament to resilience that veers from the comical to the tragic."

Los Angeles Review of Books

How to Heal Yourself When No One Else Can

"[Amy Scher is] an inspiration, not just because she teaches us how to take healing into our own hands, but because she's living proof that it works."

Pam Grout
#1 *New York Times* bestselling author
of *E-Squared* and *E-Cubed*

"Amy has seen the truth and can be a coach to all those who seek healing and authenticity. The potential resides in all of us, so read on, do not fear failure, and fulfill your potential while living an authentic life that you create and not one imposed by others."

Bernie Siegel, MD
author of *A Book of Miracles* and
The Art of Healing

"Amy Scher takes you on a guided journey to resolve emotional, physical, and energetic blockages that get in the way of true healing. You will feel like you have a loving expert coach by your side along the way."

Heather Dane
coauthor with Louise Hay of
Loving Yourself to Great Health

"Amy Scher is a voice of calm, reassuring wisdom. Her own triumph over illness is truly inspirational, but what really puts Amy in an inspirational category of her own is her warm, kind, down-to-earth, truly accessible approach."

Sara DiVello
bestselling author of *Where in the OM Am I?*

"Amy's story is awe-inspiring. Her book is full of wisdom and easy-to-implement techniques that have the power to help anyone reconnect their mind with their body and their heart with their soul and heal their entire lives. A really beautiful read."

Luminita D. Saviuc
author of *15 Things You Should Give Up to Be Happy*

"*How to Heal Yourself When No One Else Can* is a comprehensive and user-friendly DIY manifesto that's the real deal. Amy guides readers toward authentic self-healing in a way that's easily accessible, honest, and relevant for today."

Chris Grosso
author of *Indie Spiritualist*

"Amy is a courageous pioneer in the field of mind-body-spirit healing. With proven, easy-to-follow techniques, you will gain insight into the root cause of pain, physical dysfunction, and illness and transform your health. . . . This book illuminates the path to wellness."

Sherrie Dillard
author of *Develop Your Medical Intuition*

how to heal yourself
from depression
when no one else can

ALSO BY AMY B. SCHER

How to Heal Yourself When No One Else Can:
A Total Self-Healing Approach for Mind, Body, and Spirit

How to Heal Yourself from Anxiety When No One Else Can

This Is How I Save My Life: From California to India,
a True Story of Finding Everything When You Are Willing to Try Anything

how to heal yourself
from depression
when no one else can

A Self-Guided
Program
to Stop
Feeling Like
Sh*t

Amy B. Scher

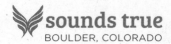

sounds true
BOULDER, COLORADO

Sounds True
Boulder, CO 80306

This book is not intended as a substitute for the medical recommendations of
physicians, mental health professionals, or other health-care providers. Rather,
it is intended to offer information to help the reader cooperate with physicians,
mental health professionals, and health-care providers in a mutual quest for optimum well-being. We advise readers to carefully review and understand the ideas
presented and to seek the advice of a qualified professional before attempting to
use them.

Published 2021

Cover design by Jennifer Miles
Book design by Maureen Forys, Happenstance Type-O-Rama
Illustrations © 2021 Richard Sheppard

The wood used to produce this book is from Forest Stewardship
Council (FSC) certified forests, recycled materials, or controlled wood.

Printed in the United States of America

Library of Congress Cataloging-in-Publication Data
Names: Scher, Amy B., author.
Title: How to heal yourself from depression when no one else can : a
    self-guided program to stop feeling like sh*t / Amy B. Scher.
Description: Boulder, CO : Sounds True, 2021. | Includes bibliographical
    references.
Identifiers: LCCN 2020025067 (print) | LCCN 2020025068 (ebook) | ISBN
    9781683646204 (paperback) | ISBN 9781683646211 (ebook)
Subjects: LCSH: Depression, Mental—Alternative treatment—Popular works.
Classification: LCC RC537 . S3838 2021 (print) | LCC RC537 (ebook) | DDC
    616.85/27—dc23
LC record available at https://lccn.loc.gov/2020025067
LC ebook record available at https://lccn.loc.gov/2020025068

10 9 8 7 6 5 4 3 2

This book is for every person
who can't *just get help*, won't *just get help*,
or did *just get help* and it didn't help.
My great hope is that this book gives
you the peace you've been looking for.

Joy sat me down and said it's time to talk, I've missed you.

—SHANNON KAISER

Contents

List of Illustrations

Where We Start:
My Story, Your Story,
Every Story

You have probably picked up this book because you are at a loss
for what to do next to help yourself. Maybe you feel so depressed
that you can barely drag yourself through a day. Or maybe you get
out of bed just fine but are experiencing life in a way that has you
asking, *What's the point of all of this?* In fact, you may feel like you're
sleepwalking, fumbling, or zoning out through life. In this day of
constant social-media bragging, motivational memes, and inspirational quotes, it's impossibly exhausting to reach that mountain of
HAPPINESS that we've all been programmed to chase (spoiler alert: it
doesn't even exist).

When we can't get to said happiness, and we're feeling like shit
because of it, we usually begin to search frantically—and I have
been no exception to that activity. When we feel bad, depressed,
or even just simply lost, we tend to rack our brains for what has
messed us up so badly. We think back upon our lives to who did
what to hurt us, what we've lost, and to all the traumas we've
endured. Before we know it, we are off and running on a full-
charge-ahead hunt for WHAT HAPPENED that sent us wildly off the
rails, ruining our life.

We look high and low, checking off everything from our list: the imbalanced chemical, the broken relationship, the stress, the nutritional deficiency. We listen to our caring doctors and focus on fixing THE THINGS THAT MADE THIS HAPPEN. We *do* a bunch of things to help ourselves feel better. We do yoga, we do therapy, we do medication. We do self-care like it's a job that our life depends on. We fix it all, and often, we still don't feel better. So we keep searching and doing. But the doing exhausts us because it's so freaking hard to do anything when you feel like you're coming undone. *Everyone else seems fine*, we think, seeing confirmation plastered all over social media. And the few of our friends who aren't fine, well, they have "been through worse" than us, we conclude. Why then, do we, maybe even having all we want, feel like life is an empty hole?

Maybe this feeling is always there for you and maybe it waxes and wanes, popping through your blue skies again and again when you least expect or understand it. Depression is something that can occur during obvious times of change and stress, after those times have settled, or rise up during what seems like the best stretches of time in our lives. Depression can happen even when you have everything you've ever wanted—when it seems that you *should* be the happiest.

But no matter when or how it happens, the inevitable question remains: *What is wrong with me?* So, on top of feeling like shit, we might also feel "not good enough." Unworthy. Ashamed. Guilty. Which was likely there long before the depression, even if you don't yet realize it.

If this whole mess sounds like the one you're in, I understand. Because this story has been mine too. And the fact that after all you've done, you still aren't cured . . . isn't actually as much of a mystery as it seems. Because it's likely that much of what you've been trying to fix is not the *entire problem*.

By my late thirties I had, finally, captured the clichéd pot of gold containing *what matters most: health.* Just a decade earlier, I had been near death with a debilitating complexity of illnesses—chronic Lyme disease, nerve damage, autoimmune conditions, anxiety, and more. Exasperated after exhausting all medical options in the United States, I traveled across the world for an experimental stem cell treatment in Delhi, India. After almost nine weeks of simultaneously drowning and thriving in my new world, I took home with me a radically changed body and—like a car that had been sitting idle, waiting for a new part—it jump-started my life. There was almost no part of me recognizable from when I'd first arrived, in a wheelchair, doped up on prescription painkillers, vying for even a chance at reaching my next birthday. But just a year after my epic adventure in India, I found myself slowly sliding backward. I was disgusted, heartbroken, and at a loss for where to turn next. While the treatment had *gotten* me healthy, it was clear I had no real foundation for sustaining that coveted title I wanted so badly: CURED. My body was, for some then unknown reason, undoing the health that medical advances had so graciously gifted me.

It was that low point in my life that opened me up to a new way of seeing things. I realized that the illness had not come out of nowhere, as I once thought—a robber in the night, to take my life without permission. Instead, I discovered that my illness was more than just the simple equation of physical malfunction = physical symptoms. Even with this epiphany that there was more to be uncovered, I had to contend with the difficult question of *What next?* Because what do you do when you've already gone around the world for the cure? It wasn't until that point that I began to connect the dots on a stretched-out map of my life—between mind *and* body. My close examination of the link between how emotional trauma and stress affect our physical

3

bodies was what opened up an entirely new path to health for me. Through the very same techniques I'm going to teach you in this book, I was able to do what no doctor or medicine could do for me: heal permanently and completely. After spending hundreds of thousands of dollars and consulting what felt like all the experts in the world, it turned out that, eventually, I had to stop chasing the cure and turn inward to address the deepest parts of *myself*. What I wish I had learned at that point, about getting to *well*—and staying there—is that it's impossible to set off to hunt down the things you need to fix and check "me" off the list forever so you can move on to happily ever after.

But I didn't know any of this after I had healed myself. During the almost ten years following my experience in India, my life felt like some kind of made-for-movie miracle. I had married my most perfect person, bought a house in Los Angeles, and built a fulfilling career helping others who were suffering just like I had. I wrote, taught, and shared everything I learned from my own healing process. I threw my life into my work, trying to build it up big and tall enough to reach every person who needed it. I had become a master at helping people detect emotional blocks, energetic causes, and subconscious thoughts that could be contributing to their symptoms or challenges. Much of my "perfect" life was driven by the will to help others—my waiting list of clients, animals that needed homes, people I knew who were going through difficult times—and everyone in between. I, however, never seemed to make it onto my own list.

By age thirty-eight, after I had finally convinced myself I had done enough to make up for all the *lost from Lyme* years of my twenties, I began to find myself tired, overwhelmed, teary, depleted, disconnected, and sometimes simply unhappy for "no reason." The previous year had been an extremely challenging one for me personally. Whether it was that year that had cast this dark shadow on me or something more subtle that had gone unidentified, it became clear that it was something I couldn't easily shake. Had I not fulfilled the requirements for true healing and happiness already, or not done it all *right* before? Was I just tired, or . . . *depressed*?

I was no stranger to depression, having grown up with a dad who, for most of my life, struggled immensely with depression. None of the various diagnoses assigned to his depressive episodes had been cured by the treatments prescribed. His struggle was heartbreaking, with erratic highs and lows, pulling our entire family along with him. And yet during my own experience with debilitating physical illness, I had never considered myself *depressed*. I had certainly felt depressed at times in my life before: during my teen years, as many of us do, and especially during my experience with debilitating illness. But it all felt circumstantial, easily explained by what I'd been going through. Now, though, when I had so much to be thankful for, I felt able to enjoy so little of it.

By the time this wave of heaviness hit, I had already been helping clients heal for years—from fatigue, depression, anxiety, illness, and more—with great success. Yet here I was, in the same position as my dad once was, and as so many of my clients had described: "having it all," "not knowing what was *that* wrong," and feeling . . . like shit.

After my dad had passed away, and with all of his wise advice gone with him, I turned to his childhood friend, Barry. Barry is the man I extract pieces of my dad from: a sliver of a memory, a funny story, and sometimes clues to what had gone wrong with him. Barry helps me piece together the father who helped me understand myself. "Barry, did Dad suffer with depression when he was young?" I asked. "I do think your dad was depressed, but we didn't talk about depression in those days," he explained. *What if they had talked?* I wondered.

It was only once I began talking to other people around me that I discovered so many others were having a hard time too. Even with "no good reason," some of them described feeling sad, bruised, apathetic, unsure, and lost. It was then that I came to a true understanding about the spectrum that we so casually refer to as *depression*. Depression is a spectrum that can range from low-grade (mild) to severe. It can be everything and anything and nothing of what it seems. Seeing depression in this new light, I scanned back over my life to realize that this may actually not be a new—or simply circumstantial—feeling for me after all.

What I realized next, about how and why I and those around me were struggling, became undeniable, irrefutable. We had lost the tether to our own core, becoming disconnected from ourselves and our lives: who we really are.

Depression is the literal *depression* of self. It happens while you are busy not meeting your own needs and, even unconsciously, are grieving for them. Depression is often born from the deep conviction that *I don't matter*. Maybe it's because you have been living for others, for your old traumas, or for that epic career you have tried so hard for. Maybe you *can't* live for you because you are buried under the stuff of your life.

For me, it became clear that my lifelong pattern of being overly sensitive to the needs and wants of others had seriously caught up to me. "Your dad was like that too," Barry said. *What if they'd talked?* I wondered again. But even more importantly, *What if we all talked?* Because it's not too late for us. The problem is that all the *doing* good we *do* for ourselves—the yoga, the meditation, the self-care, and maybe even the medication—might not be enough on its own. There is no amount of doing that will excuse us from the requirement of the deepest, toughest, and truest self-care we seek: BEING ATTENTIVE TO OUR OWN LIVES AND NEEDS.

Depression is a *side effect* of being buried under our lives and, because of that, cut off from ourselves. It is the wave that comes, either by ripple or crash, when we ignore our own needs for too long, often because it's too painful, and in favor of the demands and expectations we've created for ourselves. Sometimes, even when nothing terrible is happening, life comes just too fast and furiously to catch up to. Maybe you don't know who you are anymore, and maybe you never did. But depression is the call to let yourself rise.

If we want to close the gap of empty space within ourselves, something has to give. While it may be impossible to live a life 100 percent dedicated to what we desire, there is something more we can be doing. In addition to eliminating the noise (the trauma, the fears, and the old patterns) that blocks us from getting as close as possible to our desires, we must make an unwavering commitment to our own lives. It was this combination that helped me circle back to myself, with so many of my clients and students following right behind. The work of becoming our truest selves allows us to reach the kind of real-deal happiness that's not only attainable, but sustainable.

The medicine is not in finding *the cure*, it's in the attention to why you need the medicine in the first place. It is in learning how to stay in touch with ourselves; and how, when we lose touch, to renavigate, reposition, re-angle, and reconnect. That is what our lives—and this book—are about.

Despite all the work I had done to heal myself at the core, I was not immune to depression. I'm still not. None of us are. Depression happens because sometimes we need to be reminded that our lives require us to stay tuned in to the very purpose of them: joy.

If you have done all the doing and have corrected the things that were diagnosed as "wrong" and still aren't feeling better, there is something *else* making you feel like shit. But *you* are just fine. I know, when you feel like you do, you can't imagine anything inside of you actually being okay, but just try to trust me here. The problem is what you are buried *under*. The stuff *on top* of you—the trauma, the people, and things that have taken precedence in your life—has cut you off from yourself. *This* is the heaviness you feel. This is *depressing* you.

Your healing is doable. There's still time for you. The only thing you need to know right now is that life is not about getting *to* happiness. It's about building a bridge back to ourselves in order to allow the ease and contentment we already have. My endgame is to help *you* unbury yourself from all the stuff that's making you feel like shit so you can become the true you—the happiest, healthiest version of yourself. I want you to be able to feel good even when it's hard, when circumstances aren't perfect, and when the people around you can't help. Or even when things around you are just fine and you don't understand why *you* are falling apart.

As the motto in our house goes, *It's going to be okay and I'm going to help you.*

Let's go, my friend.

PART I

The Path:
From Feeling Bad to Good
(and Good Enough)
Discovering a New Way

Depression is not all in our head. It's not all in our body, either. Depression happens in the whole self. Depression is a condition that arises from a misalignment or disconnection in your being. As I see it, depression is not *the problem*. It's a side effect of it. But just as depression happens in the whole self, healing does too.

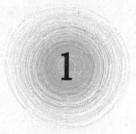

Why We Really Feel Like Shit (Even When There's "No Good Reason")

Times of feeling bad are totally normal, although many of us learned early in life to resist these feelings (which we'll fix together, soon). Life brings difficulties and challenges that we meet with all kinds of emotions: confusion, grief, sadness, frustration, anger, and more. Our moods ebb and flow, our feelings change, and more. If strong feelings remain, though, and there is no trigger or "reason" that we can identify, *depression* is often the label we end up with.

In this chapter, we're going to talk about a new way of looking at depression, from an energetic perspective. All of my insights about depression will be shared from this perspective. These do not negate any diagnosis or perspective that your health-care practitioner has shared with you. My perspective is simply an additional, and maybe new, way of seeing things. I hope this chapter will help you not only find compassion for yourself and why you are feeling bad, but also give you hope that there's so much we can still do to help you, together.

What Depression Is Really About

There are endless theories and studies about the causes of depression. While I'm not going to cover them here, what we do know now is that how we understand it is constantly evolving. One way this is true is the evolution of thinking—from our health "is all in our genes" to it's definitely "not all in our genes." The field of epigenetics, the study of how our thoughts, lifestyle, and environment switch genes on and off, has taught us that our DNA isn't the driving force behind all that ails us. You are an active player. We used to equate the body to a machine that, when malfunctioning, had a broken mechanism; we now consider that the operator (aka you) of the machine itself is just as important to look at.

In line with the old "it's the genes" school of thought, we know our current paradigm of looking for chemical, biological, or behavioral glitches doesn't offer all the answers. Based on a trend of studies, the issue of depression is getting worse, not better, despite all the drug and therapy interventions we have available to us.

I've met an endless number of people who have received this or that diagnosis and fixed it with this or that suggested solution—and still remained depressed. This was true for my own dad, who had corrected every chemical and hormonal imbalance in his brain and body with no lasting relief. But it's not all that surprising. That's because, while certain gene expressions or biochemical processes most certainly affect our bodies, we also know that our thoughts, emotions, and stress play just as significant a role.

The bottom line is clear: wherever depression comes from, the way we approach healing from it doesn't always work to the degree we want and need.

Working with the body's energy system, which we'll be doing in this book, is an entirely different way of working to heal depression—but you don't have to choose only one approach. In fact, you should most definitely not abandon whatever you are currently doing with your health-care practitioner. This is not about either/or. It can, and should, be both/and. This book is not about making a case that whatever's being done for depression is wrong. This book is about you—and knowing that if you've felt like a freak who doesn't get better after following all the leads and trying all the medications, you are not alone. These are the precise types of cases that doctors, natural practitioners, and psychologists have referred to my work for help. And I suspect that the scenarios where nothing else has worked are more the majority than has been believed. All this to say one important thing: there is something additional, and perhaps deeper, that can be done to help you feel better, and we're here to do it.

Depression can be the silent way that we grieve for our needs unmet and desires unfulfilled. It is how we *feel* the disconnection from ourselves. In fact, *depress*, by definition, means to push or press down. Over time, what we push or press down (suppress), ignore, or are unaware of becomes the weight we carry through life—our emotional "baggage." It's the stress we hold inside of us. If we carry this baggage long enough without resolution, it can over-power us and cut us off from our connection to ourselves, and thus from our inherent joy and interest in life. Emotional baggage does not cause depression but rather prevents happiness as a natural occurrence. This is a heavy burden to bear—but none of it is your fault. Let me share an analogy to help you understand how you might have gotten where you are.

How Depression Happens: Meet the Volcano

Depression is a condition that arises from a misalignment or disconnection in your being. As I see it, depression is not a singular problem. Depression is the result of the *real* problem: getting separated from ourselves, and therefore, losing our connection to life.

Depression can happen for many reasons, but *none* of them are because you are broken. You have ended up separated from yourself because of something called *life*, which comes with the traumas and complexities of being human. Eventually, all the "stuff" you've been trying to contain inside your being simply becomes too much. I liken this process to a volcano that can only contain so much pressure before it erupts, covering everything in a thick layer of sludgy lava. Depression is a result of the eruption, covering us with a thick layer of heaviness that buries us under our own lives.

Sometimes, people get depressed during a time of great distress. Sometimes, depression seems to come from "out of the blue," after a stressful event has passed, or even when everything is going smoothly. While depression can feel like it happens suddenly and for no reason, it usually happens more like a slow fog that rolls in over time; more likely, it is only the *realization* of depression that seems sudden. Sometimes the grief over our lives only comes when it's ready—when *we* are ready.

Either way, when there is enough suppressed emotional baggage stuck deep down inside of us, we often end up splitting off from our depressed pain and ourselves—without effective tools to make our way out of it. To complicate things, much of what I just described is happening outside of our awareness. That's why many people have a hard time identifying the cause of depression, or even when it might have started. This is even more true for caregivers, who while being focused on others tend to ignore their own needs.

Because our emotions are the root of who we are, everything we experience is tied to our emotional selves. And this is the part of us that is at the core of depression. In fact, your emotions drive both your biology and behavior. The late Candace Pert, a well-respected neuroscientist and the author of *Molecules of Emotion*, wrote that unexpressed emotions are literally lodged in the body, not just a product of the mind. She summed up their affect perfectly: "A feeling sparked in our mind—or body—will translate as a peptide being released somewhere. [Organs, tissues, skin, muscle, and endocrine glands], they all have peptide receptors on them and can access and store emotional information. This means the emotional memory is stored in many places in the body, not just or even primarily, in the brain." And "when emotions are repressed, denied, not allowed to be whatever they may be, our network pathways get blocked, stopping the flow of the vital feel-good, unifying chemicals that run both our biology and our behavior."[1] Our biology refers to our bodies, and our behaviors refer to our minds. Dr. Pert's statement is a perfect example of why chemicals and hormones may be imbalanced with depression, yet the depression is so often not resolved by fixing imbalances.

See the mess you've been in? And do you now understand why it's been hard to feel better no matter how hard you've tried? Don't worry, we're going to work on turning it around together. But first, let's take a closer look at how the mind and body are directly connected to depression.

The Anatomy of Depression

Depression isn't all in your head. It's not all in your body, either. It's actually in a lot of places. Feeling shitty happens in the whole person—mind, body, and energy system. This is true even if you and your doctor have identified physical or chemical contributors to how you feel. Everything is always happening in the mind-body; it's not a case of either/or. They are both, for better or worse, intricately connected. The field of psychoneuroimmunology (PNI) has documented multiple interactions of stress and the endocrine, immune, and nervous systems that impact the way we function. This reinforces how our mind-body is a cofunctioning system, which gives us great insight into more effective healing. Let's look at how both body and mind play a role in the process of depression.

Body

The human body is composed of a network of electrical impulses that run through us: our energy system. You may be familiar with the idea of energy in the body via the common diagnostic tools of EKG and EEG (reading electrical impulses of heart and brain). The foundation of Eastern medical systems is the subtle energy system—accessed by acupuncture to regulate and enhance the healthy flow of energy inside of us. These subtle energies in our bodies run through every part of us in distinct patterns: organs, muscles, glands, and more. Each and every function of our bodies interacts with this energy system, including our emotions, thoughts, and beliefs. You'll be learning a lot more about the energy system in the next chapter. But let's talk just a bit about it now to get you acquainted.

I see the energy system as an umbrella that encompasses both mind and body. When our energies are disrupted or become sluggish and blocked, we can feel it physically and/or emotionally. An imbalance or disruption in your system can create a number of sensations, such as burning in your chest, a sensation of fear, tightness in your neck, or obsessive thoughts. Symptoms in a specific area can be an indication that you are experiencing a lack of energy flow to that very part of your body due to a blockage in your energy system.

If the flow is interrupted long enough, you may even manifest a longer-term physical problem in the area or imbalances in your chemistry (controlled by all the organs and glands, which need a healthy flow of energy to function properly). Energetically, depression often manifests as physical feelings in the chest, lungs, and back. Many people struggling with grief, hopelessness, and sadness (all related to depression) tend toward respiratory infections, muscular issues in the chest and upper back, coughs, and more. In contrast, people who tend to worry experience stomachaches and digestion issues (as worry tends to affect the stomach and other related organs). Any emotional baggage can be stuck in *any* area of the body, though. Again, we look to Candace Pert and her research for a more scientific take. She explains that emotional memory is stored throughout the body and that "you can access emotional memory anywhere in the network." Pert envisioned emotions traveling in both directions, from the brain into the body, and up the body into the brain. This is important to note when we consider how chemical imbalances may be connected to depression. Pert's research helps us understand why we may be able to affect neurochemistry by working with the body's energy system.

Our energy system is interacting with the world at all times. Each and every part of our lives affects our energy system by enhancing its flow or detracting from it. If something has a negative influence on our electrical system and does not help maintain or enhance our body's energy flow, the energy system will temporarily "short-circuit," affecting the electrical (or energetic) flow running through our muscles, glands, and other organs. Some of the things that can affect our electrical system are thoughts, emotions, foods, and other substances. But, in my experience, the emotions that Pert describes as running our biology and behavior can have an equal or greater impact on us than our external environment. This is because suppressed emotions cause stress in the body, triggering a physiological response. Simply put, feeling bad comes from having bad feelings. This is why understanding the importance of the energy body in terms of the emotional connection in depression can be such a healing revelation.

Mind(s)

You may not know this, but each of us essentially has two minds, each with its own set of functions, rules, and way of perceiving the world: the conscious mind and the subconscious mind. The conscious mind is what creates. However, neuroscience has acknowledged that the subconscious mind controls 95 percent of our lives, making it our "dominant mind." The subconscious is the mind of habit and preprogrammed rules. This leaves us with a whole lot of ideas about how to fix a problem (thank you, conscious mind) but little ability to affect that actual change to get things fixed.

Your subconscious is super intelligent—so much so that it doesn't need your help with much of anything at all. It drives multiple functions in your body without you actively making them happen, such as breathing. The subconscious mind records everything that happens in our lives, including memories, emotions, and things we've learned or perceived (messages about ourselves from other people). Just like a computer, it analyzes and organizes data and creates programming that directs behavior. You don't have to do anything consciously to make this happen. Pretty cool. But on the downside, it also drives many functions of your life without you having a thing to do with it. This is, to say the least, a problem (but just for now). That's because the information and programming in your subconscious mind is primarily based on your life experiences from before the age of seven. I know you can't see me, but I'm covering my eyes in horror over here, and I bet you are too.

If your subconscious mind doesn't need your permission or input to drive behavior, and it's relying on your pre-seven-year-old-self's historical data as a basis for that behavior, then . . . we are all basically kids running around trying to act like highly functioning adults. I have to say, I was a pretty mature child, but I'd never willingly allow my seven-year-old-self to take the steering wheel of my life. Yet, that's exactly what was going on before I discovered who the real boss of me was. That's probably what's happening to you too.

If you have been sad or hopeless because you just "can't get over" whatever it is that's been going on with you, stop right now. If you've been trying to force yourself into happiness with a boot camp–like regimen of positive thinking or whatever else, just pause. If you've been trying to feel good but have not worked in alliance with your subconscious mind to make that happen, forgive yourself right now. Take a deep breath and listen to me.

When old programming runs your life, you've essentially been fighting an impossible battle. You've essentially been trying to live for and in the *now* while playing old tapes from your past. The subconscious mind is an agent of protection. It guards that data from our past and will do anything—based on that information from our inner seven-year-old—to drive us toward what it believes is *good* for us, according to its rules or programming.

Because of how awesomely powerful the subconscious mind is, you must work *with* it in order to move forward. Understanding how depression is linked to the subconscious mind, you can see why using the conscious mind alone to get happy has never worked very well, right?

Any unhealthy and outdated programming from your childhood that you are now living your life by can contribute to depression.

This is true even if you had a happy childhood. Simply put, if you are believing, reliving, interpreting, behaving, carrying, or burying anything in your past and it no longer serves you, you are likely disconnected from your naturally joyous self.

In fact, trying to force feeling good without updating our programming can unintentionally work against us, creating a sabotage effect and further depression. But you may not need me to tell you this. You may already know from experience. How many times have you insisted you'll do *x*, *y*, or *z* and then were not able to do it, perpetuating the cycle? You'll be learning how to change this in very effective ways throughout the book. But first, let's look at one of the most important components of depression there is.

What Gets You Stuck: The Freakout *Response*

When we are buried/burdened by the emotional baggage (aka the stress) of our lives—and are without the tools to unbury ourselves, we are essentially stuck in a prolonged stress response. Hans Selye, a Hungarian doctor, was the first to put explanation to the physiological changes the body experiences when humans are stressed. You might have heard this called *fight, flight, or freeze* response, but I have lovingly coined it the *freakout* response. This happens when the amygdala in the brain responds to danger before the conscious mind registers a threat. This engages other parts of the brain and the nervous system to adapt to that stress. A surge of chemicals accompanies the *freakout* response to help get us through the stressful time. This is all a very primitive process you have no control over.

Let's go over what's going on in the system when this happens so you can get a better idea of how stress affects us and why it matters. Just don't let this cause you anxiety because we are going to deal with it all together.

* Blood is directed away from the gastrointestinal tract, spleen, and other organs that are not absolutely needed to keep you alive this minute.

* The body produces additional glucose.

* Adrenal glands increase the production of cortisol and adrenaline, which, over time, can affect health.

* The immune system becomes inhibited.

* Areas of the brain related to memory and reasoning are affected (precisely why it's so hard to think your way out of stress).

* Heart rate and blood pressure increase.

* An inflammatory process gets triggered in the body as a defense/protective mechanism for danger such as infections (there is growing evidence that chronic inflammation can exacerbate or even give rise to depressive symptoms).

While your physical being drives part of the response, it is also governed by a major part of the energy system called the triple warmer meridian (an energy pathway in the body). You can think of the triple warmer meridian as an inner protective "papa bear." The triple warmer is intertwined with the nervous system, immune system, conscious mind, subconscious mind, and so much more. During the *freakout* response, energetically speaking, the triple warmer meridian (your papa bear) is on high alert, trying to fight off or keep you safe from harm.

Stress in itself is not dangerous, which you'll learn more about later, but humans have a tendency to hold the stress in our bodies and push ourselves forward instead of dealing with it effectively. In other words, once a threat passes, the brain should direct the *freakout* response to shut off (stop freaking out) so the body can move into a state of recovery. However, in our modern world where there's little "time" to process experiences, emotions, or anything else, this important recovery phase gets skipped. During the *freakout* response, your body can't handle anything but this one thing, so other nonvital biological activities are put on the back burner. This response to danger originally evolved to help our ancestors survive when they were met with threats to their physical safety—and it made great sense in those situations.

The trouble is that the body and mind cannot differentiate between an actual threat to our physical safety and stress in the form of emotional baggage (including the behaviors driven by stuff from our past). In fact, as worry-prone humans, we are often concerned about the wrong kind of stress, like how much we have to do (think chores, tasks, and our endless to-do lists) versus what we are carrying inside of us as emotional burdens. We often ignore the latter, which is precisely the kind of stress that affects our mental and physical well-being the most.

When the *freakout* dynamic is at play, your body and brain are working hard to keep you alive and safe, and as such, your programming tells you that your biological functions aren't important and also that *this is no time for change* even if it's positive. This results in getting you stuck in your current state. Our innate fight, flight, or freeze programming tells us we must concentrate only on survival, which means doing the bare minimum to get by. This translates to avoiding new regimens, behaviors, and so on, meaning we get blocked from doing the very things that would help us to feel better. This is why it is so darn hard to help yourself when you're depressed. It is not for lack of will or desire, it's because of your survival mechanism. This entire process is exactly why it's not that difficult to find yourself feeling suddenly crappy—and then once in that state, not so easy to just get out of it. And as I'm sure will be no surprise to you, this process can also lead to physical symptoms, because your body simply can't function well enough in this *freakout* state in order to keep all systems working as they should be.

When we're in stress mode, the body is essentially saying "nothing matters but survival." The *freakout* response, in an effort to protect us, often ends up keeping us not only from the help we need, but from being in touch with what matters to us at a deeper level—such as connections to family and friends, activities we enjoy, and more, which keep us fulfilled spiritually and energetically.

Being in *freakout* mode is a bad habit in the mind-body that both gets us stuck *and* keeps us stuck. You can think of it as a kind of subconscious self-sabotage. The important thing to know is that you are reprogrammable. In fact, even just doing this work is going to help toward putting you into relaxation mode.

If you're anything like I once was, the worst part of feeling bad is how out of control you feel with how you feel. This is a common complaint I hear from my clients too. But this very feeling is part of what often inspires us to participate more fully in our own healing—and what instigates some of the actual healing. By using techniques for yourself, on yourself, you are immediately changing some of what creates the fight, flight, or freeze dynamic: feeling out of control, afraid, and freaked out. If you are focused solely on a chemical imbalance, bad genes, and so on, you are triggering your own body into being and staying stuck. If you are working from the standpoint of reconnecting with yourself via self-healing, you are reversing it. Self-healing is not about having to take it all on yourself; it's about participating in your own healing in a way that sends this strong message to your mind-body: *I am okay. I am safe.*

Why Forcing Change Won't Work

Humans have the incredible ability to protect ourselves (via the fight, flight, or freeze response) and also to heal ourselves. We are complete machines that have everything we need to survive. The bummer is that human beings can't do both functions very well at the same time. That's why if you try to push or power through and treat your body like it's in boot camp, things are likely to get worse. I know you are desperate to get out of this state that you're in, but pushing furiously against where you are will not work. The fact is, radical or forced change—even change that's for the better—can cause great resistance within the body, further triggering the *freak-out*, which perpetuates the problem. And all of this feels really, really *bad*. Depressing, in fact.

While it's such a normal human reaction to try to avoid or rush through suffering, doing so only prolongs the suffering. Think back to times when you tried to avoid feeling bad or dealing with reality. Maybe that describes your whole life, like it did mine—and it's catching up to you now. No judgment. But I'm sure you can now see that fighting your reality (even while trying to change it) doesn't make anything go any faster. And it can make the "now" pretty freaking miserable. The point is that *resistance creates resistance*. The good news is that you don't have to be stress-free and in a Zen-like state in order to start healing. But you've gotta give up the fight of trying to *not* be where you already are. The energy of fighting and the energy of healing are *opposing* energies.

If you can do yourself the favor of allowing where you are to be okay (just for now) without the insistence of fixing the situation immediately, it will be far easier to start feeling better, even right where you are now.

While I'll never ask you to *like* where you are, I cannot stress enough that it's essential for you to stop hating it. Acknowledging *what is* helps calm the *freakout* response to free up your energy for change. Think of it as a smart and strategic trade. You'll never be able to fight your way to feeling better, but you can trade some of that resistance in order to flow there more easily.

In order to feel *good*, we need to help you out of *freakout* mode and into healing mode. Herbert Benson, MD, an expert in mind-body medicine, is known for coining the term "relaxation response," which is the act of turning off the fight, flight, or freeze mechanism in order to support healing. The relaxation response is what is supposed to happen—but often doesn't—after the threat of danger or a stressful event has passed. It's this element—which helps you recover from stress—that's been the missing piece all along. But, you cannot do it by fighting your way out.

The Anxiety-Depression Connection

Many people oscillate between anxiety and depression, and I have experienced this pattern myself. I see anxiety and depression as two sides of the same coin. Here's my take, which you might resonate with.

Anxiety is what may happen when we feel our suppressed emotions trying to bubble up and out of our bodies. Feeling "anxious" is the sensation that something bad is happening. What you are feeling is not necessarily bad, but it sure does feel that way. The "bad" is the energy of old emotions coming up against the resistance you have put in place to feeling your feelings (aka emotional suppression). In this state of being, you are actually tapped *into* your emotions but are not dealing with and releasing them. I find anxiety to be more common in those who tend toward the *fight* or *flight* aspects of fight, flight, or freeze.

Depression can happen with the deep disconnection from self—meaning that you are either feeling the grief of your pain, including that of your needs not being met, or are removed from what's going on inside because you are not in touch with it at all. This can leave you feeling like you are floating around without any feelings. I find that depression follows more of a *freeze* pattern of the fight, flight, or freeze response.

It's my experience that anxiety typically comes first, even if it's ignored or not recognized. And when we don't deal with it, we tend to move into more of a "depressed" state because it is simply too uncomfortable to be so highly attuned to our feelings without the resolution of them.

The Spectrum: How Depression Shows Up

Depression can be confusing and mysterious because it can show up in such different ways for different people. Depression might manifest in obvious ways like feeling sad all the time or having no interest in life, like being holed up in a house alone, being too exhausted to get out of bed, unable to socialize or go to work. But depression can also show up in such small ways that most of us who exhibit the symptoms wouldn't consider ourselves depressed: the simple lack of *umph* or gusto during the day, the sense of not knowing what we want or where to go, and not caring about things we want to care about. But the main commonality is often the feeling of *What's the point?* What I mean by this is the feeling of being drained about your situation, not seeing the other side, or why it even matters that you keep trying. In other words, feeling hopeless.

You know now that depression isn't just happening in your head. But let's talk more about the physical symptoms that can go along with depression. In fact, body aches and pains are often the first sign of depression and often what some people seek help for, even before recognizing that they also don't feel good emotionally. But symptoms can be of a wide variety, including back pain, digestive issues, fatigue, joint stiffness, and so much more. It is often indeterminable if the physical symptoms or the depression came first because our mind-body is so intertwined. We simply may notice them in one or the other initially. This can depend on your personal experiences. For example, I am highly attuned to my body because of the severe physical discomfort I endured for so long. So I tend to notice what's going on in my body before I even begin to think about how I feel emotionally. But you may be the opposite. The body and mind are windows into one another, so if we're trained to pay attention, we can interpret what's going on in one from the other. It's important to point out here that being physically ill, especially for a long period of time, can make you feel depressed. Studies show that the worse the painful physical symptoms one has, the more severe the depression tends to be.[2] That's why we'll be addressing the emotional connection to the physical body during our time together.

Because many people have absolutely none of the typical symptoms that you might imagine go along with depression as you once knew it, I want to share some ways it might show up:

* Negative, compulsive, or obsessive thoughts

* Feeling disconnected from others

* Feeling like you are at a distance from or on the "outside of" life

* Inability to relax

* Difficulty making decisions

* Being too hard on yourself (self-critical)

* Feeling shaky or unstable

* Having unexplained physical symptoms (especially fatigue or body aches)

* Feeling sad, angry, or pretty much any other difficult emotions without relief

* Being moody

* Inability to concentrate

* Extreme sensitivity around others

* Difficulty sleeping or disrupted sleep patterns

* Not caring about life, friends, or activities

* Not being able to identify your opinions or how you feel about things

* Not being able to see any "bright side" of life

* Feeling nothing (being numb)

The Silent Aspects of Depression

One of the things my clients seek to understand most is "where this came from"—and often, part of this "where" is something linked to an event or emotion from even before they were born. In other words, you may have had some of it all along. I don't tell you this so that you feel delicate or irreparable. Neither of these things is true. I tell you this so that you can have a complete understanding of why you might feel how you feel. This has no bearing on your healing outcome.

There are two dynamics that we often aren't aware of that can contribute to depression (and, thankfully, contribute to healing when addressed): energetic sensitivity and inherited energy. When we look at these dynamics in terms of depression, it is not only your own "stuff" that's creating a disconnect between you and yourself, but other people's stuff too. I joke with my clients about this, telling them we have enough of our own shit, we don't need to be carrying everyone else's too. All kidding aside, while these energies are important to pay attention to, I don't usually find they are impacting a person more than their own energies. In other words, integrate working on these in your process, but don't let them distract you from focusing on everything else.

You will be working on inherited energy in part IV of the book, where you learn next-level approaches. You will be working on energetic sensitivity throughout this book, including in part IV. Let's go over them each a little bit more.

Energetic Sensitivity

I often hear people who are depressed say they are "sensitive," have a hard time just being in the world, are affected by everything and everyone, and feel like life is tougher or more overwhelming for them than it is for those around them. On the flip side, others might describe these same people as *the rock*, the person who can make anyone feel better, or the one who "has it all under control." If you find yourself exhausted, sad, tired, drained, anxious, or devoid of joy while simultaneously lifting everyone else up, you may be what's called an empath—meaning you are likely "energetically sensitive"—and the energy of those around you has a great effect on you. Because the nervous system acts as our antenna for the world, highly empathic people simply pick up on and are more tuned in to emotions than others may be. This phenomenon is very common in natural caretakers.

The truth is that some of us simply come into this world as sensitive beings, which, in turn, can create a heightened sensitivity to stress, other people's emotions, and the world at large. But as someone who has had to work through this myself, I can absolutely say that being energetically sensitive is so much more than just being born that way. And it can be hugely improved so it doesn't affect you negatively—but it takes more than doing exercises to "protect" yourself (although they can't hurt, for sure). Here's why.

Energetic sensitivity can happen as a response to unresolved trauma. Having our own emotional baggage makes it much easier to "match up to" or relate deeply and energetically to other people's stuff. If you think back, you may have been most affected by the world around you when you yourself were going through hard times. That's because in your own state of heightened sensitivity or emotional pain, we can end up more tuned in to that in others. In addition, energetic sensitivity is absolutely directly tied to your ability to say *no* in life: your boundaries. Energetic sensitivity is amplified when we don't consciously set the distinction between *us* and *other*. You will never be able to do enough protection exercises to feel better. In other words, you have to deal with your own stuff, too, which will help strengthen your entire energy system. You're going to do this by healing emotional baggage (part II of this book) *and* drawing boundaries (chapter 8).

Your sensitivity has many positive aspects. I don't want you to see it as a curse. But we want to make it work for you, not overwhelm you. The worst thing you can do is dive into it, start being afraid of the world around you, and surrender your powerful self. It's simply a hiccup in the system that we can work with.

Inherited Energy

I often work with people who feel heavy or depressed and remember it always being this way. In the same way we get many of our parents' personality traits and physical characteristics, we can also take on some of the energy of our parents. This means we all have what's called inherited or generational energy. Some of us have lineages where family members have experienced great trauma or adversity. Actually, this is true for most of us. The field of epigenetics has been closely studying how our ancestors' trauma may affect our lives and biology. My own family members were survivors of the Holocaust, which I believe is heavily woven into my family's energetic fabric. If you had parents, grandparents, or other relatives who experienced great trauma, you may especially resonate with this. This means we are carrying not only our own "stuff" but also that of our ancestors. This inherited energy can affect your life in the same way your own stress does, which means energy from your ancestors may be getting in the way of your truest, most joyful self.

A sign that you are experiencing this phenomenon is feeling like you've always had a black cloud over you that you can't identify a point of origin for. Sometimes, you'll see a pattern in your family where everyone is struggling, but for some reason, it's more often just a couple of other people in your family who are being negatively affected by inherited energy. Either way, this is a great opportunity for you. My clients report that clearing inherited trauma and energy is extremely cathartic. Because it's been passed from generation to generation, it can feel very "heavy" to carry but be so very freeing to let go of.

No matter how you experience depression or why it's there, it's likely your body's way of telling you that all of what you've been carrying and how you've been living life is not working for you.

And after a very long time of maybe not knowing where to turn, understanding even just that is the only start we need.

You may be feeling a little bit overwhelmed with all of the moving pieces that we've talked about here. But we're going to be doing the healing together. Piece by piece. And there is no right way to address it, or need to do it all or all at once. Phew.

It has been my life's work to put all the pieces together to help people just like you move from feeling bad to feeling good (and good enough), even when nothing else has helped before. You're next.

Let's learn about my energetic healing approach so you can see how this is all going to work.

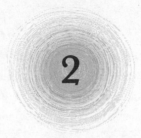

2

A Brand New Approach:
Energy Therapy

You understand now that depression can be a form of grieving. You also understand why you can't overcome depression with willpower or positive thinking: because most of what causes feeling bad is *bad feelings*. And not all those feelings are in your head. Or in your genes. Depression is in your whole body and your energy body too. That's why being happy is so beyond a willful act of *being* or *thinking* happy. And we know that forcing things (as in willpower and positive thinking) often only makes things worse. This is why we need another way.

In this chapter, I'm going to outline what we'll be doing in this book and how you can benefit greatly from doing this work.

Address the Root of Depression

Many ancient medical systems focus on treating the human being instead of just the isolated "ailment" or complaint. True healing does not come from pointing to and working with just the symptom. True healing comes from changing the terrain in which the ailment rooted itself and found a home in: you.

This whole book in one way or another is about emotions— because of them *and* in spite of them, we, and depression, exist. The limbic system (the part of the brain that deals with emotions), which includes the amygdala, is what triggers the *freakout* response. It also controls the response from your autonomic nervous system in relationship to emotional stimuli and is involved in reinforcing behavior. With this in mind, you can see why focusing on emotions has a huge role in healing depression, even if you do have diagnosed chemical imbalances or other physical contributors. But depression is not just about our feelings and what's going on in our brain, because how we feel, who we are, and how we respond to the world are also intricately connected to our body's unique *energy system*. This energy system—which each and every human being has—plays a major role in how we function. That's why talking about feelings or trying to control emotional responses doesn't typically transform your life. We're often only touching upon the surface of depression when we do that.

The subtle energy system is made up of several subsystems, including chakras, meridians, and auras. The energy (referred to as *qi*, *prana*, and other names depending on the medical system and culture) gets delivered to all parts of our body and brain via energy "pathways," or patterns. In my approach, we will be moving energy throughout the entire system but often targeting only the meridians and chakras. But because all of the parts of your energy system are integrated, we'll be able to affect the entire system in a positive way even without addressing each part individually.

Sensitive practitioners of healing modalities, and even some tools, have now been able to detect imbalances in the energy system before physical or emotional symptoms occur. If the imbalance came before the "problem," it makes sense why going back to the energy system to heal it at its core is hugely effective. This is why using energy therapy often works when nothing else does. You'll be learning more about the specific parts of the energy system when you learn the techniques in chapter 3.

The general term for my work is called energy therapy or energy healing, but the more specific type of practice I utilize is called energy psychology: a group of techniques that address the relationship between the energy system *and* emotions, thoughts, and behavior. Because of this complete approach, energy therapy often works when nothing else has. The Association for Comprehensive Energy Psychology (ACEP) reports more than 100 studies (fifty-plus randomized controlled trials and fifty-plus pre-post outcome studies) with all but one documenting the effectiveness of energy psychology. Each year, more evidence emerges about the exciting benefits of this field of work.

My approach, which you'll be learning about in detail shortly, will help you do something you likely haven't done yet—address the root of depression from an emotional *and* energetic standpoint. As you learned in the previous chapter, emotions are the root of who we are, affecting both our biology and our behavior. But there's something important you need to know: emotions are the *first* domino in a series of responses in the body and brain that lead to mental and behavioral shifts. What this means is that by working with the emotional baggage stuck in the body before we try to consciously force change in how we feel, we are working in the natural order of how the body's processes work. If we try to first start with the mental aspect of ourselves and look to positive thinking, analyzing patterns, behavioral changes, and more, we are fighting an uphill battle.

Using the techniques I'm going to teach you will not only help you identify and release root emotional issues (even if they are in the subconscious mind) but also allow you to slowly make changes that recover or uncover your happiest, healthiest self. By doing this, we offer a remedy to the person and not just the ailment.

If you are familiar with my work, it may be because you have read my previous *How to Heal Yourself When No One Else Can* books, which cover how to use my unique approach to access the energy body to address energetic causes of physical illness and emotional challenges such as anxiety. While the techniques and general approach in this book are like my previous books, *How to Heal Yourself from Depression When No One Else Can* shows you the path to specifically target the energetic root of depression. In simple terms, it will help you go from feeling like shit to feeling good (and good enough). Throughout the entire process, you'll be working with energetic blocks that cause emotional *suppression* and may be contributing to *depression* at a deep level. I am going to walk you through releasing what's been holding you back and help you make changes to reconnect to yourself and your life again—or maybe, for the first time ever.

The energy system is our way *in* to unbury you from the volcano we talked about earlier. In other words, we're going *in* to get you *out*. The techniques are simply the vehicle that we'll use. While my approach is not a substitute for medical or psychiatric care, my techniques have often worked when other interventions have not. I do not attribute this to something special I'm doing that no one else is. I attribute it to the effectiveness of addressing both the mind and body (including the energy body) and to the powerful benefits of self-healing. The gentle process you're going to learn in the coming chapters is the same one that I've taught thousands of everyday people to do—people like myself who had little patience, a frustration with the standard approaches to dealing with emotions, and no desire to regurgitate all my old wounds in order to feel better. This book will not ask you to focus on and dissect what is wrong, but rather touch upon it in a way that helps you let it go, for good.

A NOTE FOR CAREGIVERS AND FAMILY MEMBERS

For those of you who are primary caregivers for loved ones or even for your profession, I see you. It is a difficult job you have in supporting someone you care for—while also trying to care for yourself. Watching someone struggle while maintaining your own balance is not easy, but it is necessary.

Depression is a heartbreaking issue not only for those suffering but also for those of us who love them, and whose own mental health often gets put on the back burner. In fact, according to the Caregiver Action Network, a Washington, DC-based nonprofit, 40 to 70 percent of family caregivers have their own clinically significant symptoms of depression.

My work regularly helps caregivers overcome the trauma and impact of mental illness in a family and reclaim their own sense of self and joy. So while you might be reading this to help someone else, please remember that this work is for you too.

My approach offers you a modernized way to integrate centuries-old wisdom and energetic healing along with today's promising field of energy psychology in order to get you feeling better. By using energy psychology, we can affect you as a whole person, shifting your perception of life's experiences, perspectives, and reality. Because our lives are filtered through our emotions, as we transform them it's likely you'll gain immediate new perspectives or feel positive shifts even if you can't change certain things about your life that you dislike. By making peace with our emotions, we can often change our perspective to feel less stressed or upset about our overall situation.

This process isn't about reaching for anything epic, although it might feel epic from where you stand now. The ultimate goal of all the work during our time together will be not to manage depression, but to find out what it's all about and then pull you out of it.

My Three-Step Approach

You'll remember that Candace Pert described how when our emotions are repressed, our network pathways get blocked, which then affects our biology (bodies) and behavior (minds). My approach addresses these angles. Through the healing process, we will be affecting all of you—body and mind(s) (conscious *and* subconscious)—all together. But we're going to take it slow and keep it simple because that's how we'll be most effective. Our focus will be on making shifts to create momentum instead of a radical overnight transformation. This approach creates change in the right direction, without causing more of the stress that leads to depression.

Together, we'll be going through these simple steps.

Step 1: Get Unstuck

Because the energy in the body runs in patterns and the fight, flight, or freeze (aka the *freakout*) response is its own pattern, stuckness can actually become the automatic go-to response in your system. Which means depression lends itself to the habit of being depressed. No wonder it's been so hard to get out, right? But trying to overcome depression by going straight into addressing deepseated emotional patterns can backfire. This is because starting too "big" when you're stuck can cause the body to resist any big moves that feel unsafe. In Step 1, we'll focus on what I call *micro movements*—to sneak the body out of its *freakout* pattern before we start doing the deeper healing work.

You'll start working on getting unstuck at the end of this chapter.

Step 2: Heal Yourself (Release Emotional Baggage)

In Step 2 we'll start digging you out by sifting through and releasing emotional baggage (aka stress). Using various techniques, we'll focus on dealing with your feelings, clearing harmful beliefs, and healing trauma from your past. This will all be essentially reprogramming your subconscious mind and body for feeling good.

You'll be working on Step 2 throughout part II in the book.

Step 3: Create Lasting Change (Addressing Life Patterns)

Finally, we are going to address patterns to create lasting change. I am sure this is not the first time someone has suggested you "change" to change your life. While that guidance is not without merit, it's also useless. Because as you now understand, your emotions are what drives your biology and behavior. And those patterns affect the quality of your life, thus creating more emotional baggage and trauma. That's why we can't always "just change" so easily, unless we've taken care of the healing first. So in Step 3, you'll be ready to learn how to listen to your body and its messages, draw your boundaries, and commit to yourself in order to create lasting change.

You'll be working on this in part III of the book.

In part IV, you'll get to take everything you've learned to the next level by learning how to customize your healing. You'll not only clear more from each topic we cover in the first parts but also target very specific symptoms, challenges, and energies that are unique to your individual situation.

My Only Rule: Do the Work

We are going to cover a lot. But don't let it overwhelm you. You do not need to do it all, or all perfectly, to start feeling better. In fact, one of my favorite sayings (by Voltaire) is relevant here: "Perfect is the enemy of good." My only rule for this work is that you have to do it and own it as yours. That's how you're going to get the most out of this process.

We are going to work on helping you shift to a better-feeling place as quickly as possible. But we're also going to honor the fact that maybe you've been stuck for a long time, and, as we talked about, it can actually stall you to try to furiously dig yourself out overnight.

I suggest keeping a dedicated notebook to use as we work together. This will help give you a place to write down notes or ideas of things to address as we go along. It will also help you feel like you don't have to rush, because you'll know it's all right there laid out for you to do, bit by bit.

Most importantly, you don't need to try to "complete" each section before moving on to the next. It will be impossible to complete this work in a tidy checklist format. Trust me, I've had many people

try (and I was one of them). Part of the healing process is actually
about learning to relax, lighten up on yourself, and keep going no
matter what—even when things feel messy. Just integrate as much
as you can from each chapter and proceed. But at the same time,
keep working on all that you have learned. If you allow yourself,
you'll find an intuitive process that leads you to working on what
you need to, at the right time. As you move through the book, continue incorporating whatever you can from previous chapters into
your life.

I want to say this one more time, because it's so worth repeating: I really, really don't want you to focus on "doing it all" or
"getting it all right." And it's absolutely not necessary to "fix it all"
in order to heal. I certainly didn't check every single issue off my list
before I was able to be happy. As a matter of fact, if I succeed in
my mission, you will be ready to leave the stressful idea of perfectionism behind for good. I just want you to keep going.

My clients and readers who've made the biggest transforma-
tions are those who have taken this work as their own, weaving
it into the fabric of their lives. This has personally been the most
rewarding part of doing and teaching the work for me. I often find
myself thinking, *I can't believe I ever lived without this stuff!* Since having
this work in my life, I truly can't imagine life without it. Sometimes
my students, friends, and family and I say to each other, "So, what
did we do before this? Just feel sick and stuck all the time?" And
the answer is, *um, yes!* Now, when something feels off or I don't
feel great, and can't figure out why, I simply use the process you're
about to learn and am able to move on.

I think you'll find that it's the coolest feeling to be able to reach
your own state of real-deal happiness (not the social-media version
we can never get to!) and then sustain that shift you've worked so hard
for. I see this work as a lifestyle of paying attention to yourself and

your needs (and attending to them when you need to, at last). The final part of this book is going to make sure you have every single way of doing that so you never have to feel stuck or hopeless again.

How This Book Is Organized

I have made my three-step approach as easy as possible for you. In the remainder of part I, you'll learn the techniques and begin getting unstuck with some super simple practices. Then, I'll guide you through exercises in parts II and III together to cover the different aspects of healing we're working on. After that, there is more you can choose to do to go even further in your journey.

Part III will get you through much good healing based on the common blocks I find with most of my clients who experience depression. I'll be with you every step of the way. In part IV, I'll offer you next-level approaches so that you can go beyond the main healing approach we do together. This is where, when you're ready, you're going to customize this work to you and master how to release any additional energies that might be keeping you stuck.

Part IV will also help you see the true diversity in my approach and techniques so you feel empowered in every way. I want you to be able to use all of the aspects of my approach quickly and efficiently as part of your consistent self-care and attention to the importance of your own life.

What to Expect

Starting a new process can create excitement, but it can also be daunting and terrifying. You might already be thinking, *This won't work*. We'll be covering this common way of thinking when we work with beliefs; but for now, try your best to stay curious and open.

Curiosity is one of the tricks for getting ourselves through times of doubt or resistance to things that will be good for us. I'm not going to ask you to be all-in from the start and convinced that this *will* work, but you can't be married to the belief that it won't, either. Instead, be curious about *how* it might work, what it might feel like, and what you'll discover. This opens you up to possibility, which is equivalent to the energy of hope. And that's a darn good place to start from.

Let's go over what you can expect during our time together.

How to Begin

I often get the very same questions about healing and writing—how do you begin? What's your process? How do you set up your space? And the list goes on. My answer is always, boringly: I've learned the hard way that the only way to do it is to do it. Healing happens by doing the work. The end. This is the same way my books get written (by writing them). If you find yourself making big plans about doing the work, setting up your space, and more, that's because you're resisting simply doing it. Keep it simple. All you need is a place to sit down or lie down. I sometimes do my energy work sitting on my bed, sometimes in the car, lying down in my yard, or in the two-minute break I take from writing to run to the bathroom. There are zero rules for how, when, and where. But there is no way around this: if you want to get from point A to point B, you have to walk there—even if it's only one step or five minutes a day.

How Energy Therapy Feels

As you use the techniques, you might experience sensations such as a temporary and sudden exhaustion (like you've hit what I refer to as the "jet lag wall" after a long trip), yawning, burping, getting the chills, stomach gurgling, sneezing, runny eyes and nose, and even something more desirable like a surge of energy or positivity. For me, I tend to yawn uncontrollably and joke that when I sneeze, it's so powerful that it counts for ten yawns. But each of us has our own feeling when we shift. Some of us don't feel anything at all, and that's perfectly alright too.

As you practice some techniques, you may notice that you can't "pay attention" and your mind is wandering to your to-do list. This is totally fine. It might be a sign that there are energies associated with those thoughts that your body is trying to release. But also, because all of the techniques incorporate the subconscious release aspect, it often means your conscious mind gets bored (because in a way, it's being bypassed). So sometimes the distracted thoughts simply mean that the process is working. If you start out very attentive and emotional but "lose interest" or care once you've been using the technique for a bit, it can also mean that you have successfully changed your reaction to it or released the stress of that energy. But I'll be guiding you through each exercise and giving you tips along the way.

Are There Any Negative Side Effects?

Sometimes, as we become aware of and work on all we've been buried under, we can feel temporarily "worse." This is not actually a reality of feeling worse but rather the reality of finally *feeling*, recognizing, or admitting what's been stuffed deep down inside of you. In other words, "the yuck" may be closer to the surface as you work with it.

Additionally, when moving and releasing old energy, people sometimes feel what's called "processing" or "recalibrating." This just means you are moving energy—yay! That's exactly what we're trying to do, so this is good news. Processing is equivalent to regaining your equilibrium when you've been thrown off. Imagine almost tripping and then stumbling a little before you get your footing back. The processing (aka the "wobble") that you might get with energy work happens as your body releases the old energy completely from your energetic field. It can manifest in any way, but some common responses are being more emotional for a day or two, feeling more tired, or feeling "off." If your symptoms are linked to processing, they will never last more than a few hours or, at the most, a few days. You can use the exercises you'll learn later in this chapter to help you feel better, faster.

Time Needed

You don't need to do this work for hours a day or in big leaps. Consistency is key. This is not a therapy you show up to once a week and then forget about in between. This work is a process you *live*. It should become part of your life, to support you but not take it over. Remember, we're working toward a new lifestyle of paying attention to yourself and your needs versus putting in endless hours trying to fix things. Because you are working on clearing away old (and sometimes very embedded) energetic patterns and retraining your system, you are going to need to show up over and over in order to set a new pattern. And probably more often at first. For example, I now use this work several times a week in short spurts to clear out anything I feel has gotten stuck in order to prevent things from piling up as they did in my past. But in the beginning, I did have to spend more time on the work because there was much more to work with. Again, this doesn't mean anything epic in terms of time or super hard work. It's about commitment and baby steps. You do have to be consistent, but you also know that you're not going to be able to "boot camp" yourself into feeling better. You also can't heal while focusing for hours a day on what's wrong (and many people don't have the luxury of that kind of time to dedicate to their healing anyway). None of that is good for you. That's not healing. That's not doable for the average person just trying to hold himself or herself together.

As a general recommendation: I suggest using the techniques in this chapter daily in very short spurts of time. I also recommend setting aside twenty or thirty minutes a few times each week to do the deeper healing work outlined in parts II and III of this book. If you have an hour or more, great! But the amount of time you spend isn't as important as what you do within that time. With all that said, you will find a rhythm that works best for you. No perfection required. Anything goes, as long as you do the work, and do it consistently.

How to Gauge Results

Some people see exciting results right away (sometimes even within a few hours or days), and some take a lot longer. If you are like me, you may not see the results you are looking for right away. I joke with some of my clients how envious I am of them for seeing improvements so quickly while I'm sitting there twiddling my thumbs, waiting for change to come!

Generally speaking, results can go from a dramatically improved feeling like "I feel like a huge cloud just lifted from my life" to "I feel just a little bit more hopeful." Typically, results are not linear, which means you can feel up and down until you feel better consistently. For me, one of my very worst months of symptoms came just before I turned a corner and everything shifted for the better. Thank goodness I didn't give up!

Because we are so used to searching for *the cure*, we often miss the more subtle signs that we are heading in the right direction. A doctor once told me that she considered even a 1 percent improvement to be a great sign of healing—especially if it comes after no improvement for a long period of time. And while inside I was screaming *I just want to be fixed!* I later saw the significance of these tiny wins. They add up.

Here are some signs of subtle healing to keep an eye out for:

You start to feel better or worse. While feeling exactly the same for long periods of time means something is stuck, feeling "worse" temporarily can be a sign that you are *moving* energy. Of course, check in with your doctor about any new signs or symptoms. But energetically speaking, any movement is good. Eventually, we want the energy to move out of your body. But even getting it to shift a little can mean we've uprooted it.

You have a more hopeful view or see the same situation in a new way. Many times, as we clear energy, what comes first are cognitive shifts (aka aha moments such as "Oh, I get why I've been feeling this way" or "Now I suddenly see what needs to change"). These cognitive shifts can allow us to see things in a new or different light, even though nothing in our circumstances has changed. This can bring a lot of relief to a current situation while we are moving the *depressed* energy that contributed to our situation in the first place. It's also often a sign that another level of changes is coming.

You are excited by the process of healing rather than daunted as before. This is a signal that you are harnessing some of your vital energy again. This is the "energy for life" we lose when we are so depressed. So feeling it again in even the tiniest way is a great sign.

You find yourself thinking about plans for your life again. Even if you aren't taking action, even daydreaming about doing things you used to do or want to do is a great shift. Again, this shows that some of your vitality is emerging once again.

Whether you see quick and dramatic results or follow in my footsteps of slower and subtle change, I assure you that your individual process or pace has no impact on your final healing outcome.

Living with any level of depression is hard. And when you feel depressed, it is even harder to help yourself, no matter how much you try. But with this book as your guide, I know you can do it.

We're now ready for our first step, getting unstuck. Then, you'll learn the basics of my signature deep healing techniques, which we'll use throughout the rest of the book to release emotional blocks that are contributing to depression.

The Secret Sauce: Micro Movements

You already understand why trying to make huge changes could backfire, overwhelming and creating even more resistance within your system. For this reason, before we do the deep work necessary to release the original causes of why you feel like shit, we'll start by getting your system to chill the heck out. Even just a little bit is going to help big-time for the long haul. Our goal is to make your body feel as safe and relaxed as possible, as consistently as possible, to gently convince the triple warmer meridian ("papa bear") that it's safe to let you out of *freakout* mode so you can live your life. Once we get toward the end of our work together, we will talk about making some important changes for your life (which you'll be able to make with much more ease once you're in a different place energetically).

If we make tiny changes, which I call micro movements, we can almost trick the body into shifting to a better place. It's a little bit of a stealth maneuver . . . but it works. Starting super small with changes can be such a game changer at this stage. Let me tell you a little story to explain.

"Take him va a long valk," is what my grandpa used to suggest eagerly over the phone in his heavy Yiddish accent. When my dad was in his depressive episodes, the people who never saw him in that state, like my grandpa, who lived across the country, had plenty of ideas about how to fix it. My grandpa had survived the Holocaust, the atrocities of which most of us couldn't even begin to grasp. Yet, he lived a life full of joy. The understanding that someone—my dad—could be depressed, with no obvious reason to speak of, escaped him. My dad was born in a displacement camp following the Holocaust, in Germany. That, along with being temporarily separated from his parents because of a medical condition as a baby, had a great impact on his life. But it still didn't seem to explain his constant struggle, especially despite the best therapies and medications then available. Almost everyone who offered ideas would suggest getting my dad to "snap out of it" in one way or another—"a walk" being the number-one recommended activity to do this with. For me, the idea seemed preposterous. It was often impossible to even get him to speak, let alone get outside the walls of our house. In my indignation, I deemed the advice useless, concluding, *No depressed person ever jumped up to take a walk and felt better.*

It was during my own illness experience that I realized, while walks aren't any kind of cure, even the smallest movement of any kind really can help. Why? Because it creates a shift in the right *direction*. And from that shift, it's easier to go a little more and a little more. The habitual patterns of our bodies, energy systems, and environments run deep. They don't budge easily. Yet still, we are humans, longing for movement and flow. Sometimes we just need help to get there: a subtle shift of energy can be the momentum we need to start.

This is often how I made progress through my own illness: by making one small movement at a time. If I could muster the energy to even change rooms where I slept most of the day, it would often help. Because my specialty now is working with clients who have chronic conditions, I've long practiced helping clients make tiny movements of their own, even in their most desperate, delicate states. *Can you maybe at least change position in bed?*, I ask, conscious not to sound like my grandpa. *Can you find one thing to do today for five minutes to distract you from your desperate thoughts?* For the record, I've still never once suggested a long walk.

But if I can at least get them talking, and maybe even laughing (a goal of mine, always), there's a lot we can do just from that tiny shift. It is not the entire healing we need in an instant, but it is a start.

It turns out my grandpa knew what he was talking about, even if it didn't seem that way at the time. What he was trying to say was SHAKE SOMETHING UP. This is what we are going to do with energy work—create a tiny bit of space and momentum to get you moving in the right direction. It's easier to feel a little better when you feel a little better. And when you feel a little better, you're more likely to see the solutions, insights, and perspectives that will help you. Just as no depressed person ever jumped up for a long walk, no depressed person ever thought his or her way out of depression either. All healing is about getting unstuck—and it's a matter of small movements that add up to the whole. You can't go from depressed to happy. You can't go from exhausted to energetic. But you don't have to.

This book will help you at just the right pace, but let's start now with showing your body that it's safe to begin.

Getting Unstuck: Exercises to Shift Your Energy

Keeping in mind that you may be *so* stuck that everything feels like
a huge leap, I am going to give you some practical and simple ways
to help create the tiniest bit of momentum. Luckily, you are learning
from the most impatient person ever—which means none of the
techniques I'm going to teach you will require a lot of time or concen-
tration. Because if they did, I never would have been able to use them.

When you practice the following exercises consistently, you are
actually retraining your body into a new way of being. With these
exercises, you are sending a message to your system of *Hey, we're going
to try this new and healthier thing now instead of that thing we've been doing
that's been keeping us stuck.*

It used to be widely believed that it took twenty-one to thirty
days to create a new habit. However, more recent information is very
telling about why so many of us fail. Researchers from the University
College London have found that the average number of days it takes
to get a new pattern to stick is sixty-six—but it can be up to 254 days
(nearly nine months!) for some people. The exact number of days it
takes you to set a new pattern doesn't matter, but the consistency and
commitment does. So if it seems like it's not working, keep going;
and if it seems like it is, do the same.

Daily Exercise: Tap + Breathe + Trace

The Tap + Breathe + Trace exercise is one I created by combin-
ing a shortcut of my Alternate Temple Tapping technique (you'll
learn it in the next chapter), some basic breath work, and one of
my favorite ways to calm the fight, flight, or freeze mechanism in
the body. Even doing these each individually is quite powerful, but
together they work like magic.

You will be using the following exercise two times per day, preferably at regular intervals (aim for morning and evening) to get the repetition and consistency we need to set a new pattern. The technique has three parts, and you'll be doing the first two for two minutes each and the last part for one minute (for a total of five minutes each session). Easy! You are free to do more, of course. But those five-minute spurts are enough for a great start. I suggest you set your phone timer to keep track.

Step one: You are going to tap on your temples for two minutes straight, alternating between temples (for example, you tap your right temple with three or four fingertips on your right hand, then tap your left temple with three or four fingertips of your left hand, switching between one temple and the other). This will quickly form a nice rhythm once you get started. Just gently tap at a pace that feels natural for you. Because the temples are where the triple warmer meridian begins, tapping on them can help release the "stickiness" that comes from being in *freakout* mode. And it's so simple and calming to do. You don't need to think about anything in particular while you're tapping, but if you focus on the things you're worried, stressed, or feel bad about during that time, the tapping will help release the worry from your system.

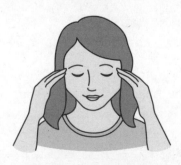

Temple Tapping Points

Step two: Once you are done with two consecutive minutes of alternate tapping, you are going to switch to two minutes of breathing. You'll do this by slowly and deliberately inhaling through your nose for four seconds, then exhaling through your mouth with pursed lips (as if you're whistling) for eight seconds. Concentrate on the feeling of breath as it comes in and out of your nose/mouth. You'll repeat this for the next two minutes.

Step three: Finally, you're going to use my adapted version of an exercise I learned from energy medicine pioneer Donna Eden, author of *Energy Medicine*. Her *triple warmer smoothie* works to release excess energy from the triple warmer meridian by tracing a portion of it backward, on the head and neck. I've added another element to engage the remainder of the meridian (down the arms) to further soothe the body's stress response. Place your hands against either side of your head so your fingertips are resting on your forehead and your palms are resting over your temples. Next, slowly and deliberately "trace" around your ears (using your flat hands, stay in contact with your head), pulling them down the sides of your neck until you reach your shoulders. This should mimic how you might "smoothe" a child's hair back from their face to calm them when upset. Now, lift your hands off your shoulders and cross your arms so that each hand is resting on the opposite upper arm. Pull your hands all the way down your arms until you reach your wrists; then immediately bring them back to the top of the arms and pull them down again a few more times (as if you are petting yourself). You'll want to use the entire sequence—starting at your temples again and ending at your wrists—for about a minute. It can be helpful to repeat an affirmation such as "I am safe" as you use this, but it's not necessary.

You may repeat this Tap + Breathe + Trace cycle as many times as you'd like, but keeping it to five minutes is totally fine. And if you need to start with a shorter amount of time and build up, that's okay too. Just remember you want to do this *twice a day*. It's also a great routine to use throughout the day when you need some extra support or calming.

Now, let's learn a couple more exercises for your toolbox.

As Needed: SOS Techniques

Because it's sometimes nice to have more tools than you need, I want to give you a few extra exercises that will be helpful in the process of getting your body to go from *freakout* to chill-out (aka getting you unstuck). The following three exercises are all beneficial and very easy to use, even when you're feeling at your worst. In fact, this is when they are best used. I think of them as energy therapy first aid. They are excellent to have as a go-to for when you need to calm or shift your body, but the bonus is that over time, they can help reprogram your body into a more balanced state. Use them in addition to the Tap + Breathe + Trace or whenever you are feeling extra panicked, depressed, or just stuck.

Acupoint ear rub: Because there are so many acupuncture points (corresponding to your energy system) in your ears, rubbing your ears is a very effective calming and balancing technique to help move stuck energy and reset your body. It's my favorite thing to do when it feels impossible to get out of bed in the morning as it takes almost no energy or motivation.

How to: Simply massage both ears fully (outside and inside) in little circular movements with your fingertips. There is no specific pattern you need to follow for this. Essentially you are trying to stimulate your meridians and balance your energy system by covering the entire surface of the ear and earlobes.

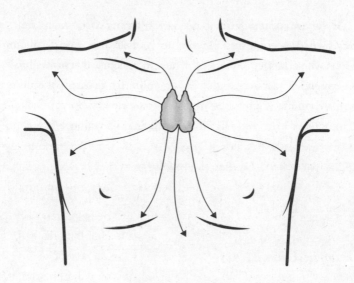

Thymus Gland

Thymus tapping: Because the thymus gland, the master gland of your immune system, is connected to the entire energy system, it can work as a stress modulator when stimulated. You might notice that you naturally touch or rub the area around your thymus gland—located behind your breastbone—when you feel anxious or upset.

Gorillas in the wild thump this area to "rev" themselves up to meet danger or signal their strength. These actions seem to be a natural tendency to strengthen and balance our energy when we need it most. In fact, this area is widely referred to as the "happiness point." Tapping the thymus gland using your fingertips is a powerful technique to help relieve stressful emotions. You'll be learning a lot more about tapping the thymus gland when you learn my technique Thymus Test and Tap in the next chapter. But for now, I'll teach you a shortcut.

How to: Momentarily focus on something that's bothering you (a worry, something a person said to you, or any single feeling like "sad" or "angry"). Now tap your thymus gland repeatedly as you say "let go, let go, let go," giving your system the opportunity to move emotions and stress out of your body to help you into a calmer, more balanced place. With tapping, you can use a few fingertips and tap with medium pressure or use your flat hand to tap against your chest. Tapping the thymus is so cool because you can release emotional stress, stimulate and strengthen your immune system, *and* calm your body all at the same time.

Helpful Checklists

When we're feeling our worst, even the "obvious" ways to take care of ourselves can easily escape us. So, in addition to the energy therapy practices, it might be helpful to have some practical ideas to guide you too.

Here are some simple checklists that will help you with daily concrete self-care rituals that create healing momentum as well.

Daily Basics

○ Fill up a water bottle to drink throughout the day.

○ Open the blinds and windows in your house (or at least in the room you sit in most) and make your bed.

○ If you have medications or supplements you take, take them all out in the morning and put them in a little dish. Keep them close to you to make them easier to take.

○ Reply to texts or emails only as you're able. If the task feels overwhelming, create one simple response message and copy and paste it to various recipients.

○ Shower or change your clothes. If you can't get dressed for the day, put fresh pajamas on.

Healthy Activities

○ Do a tiny bit of something you love. For example, if you love drawing, commit to just taking out your supplies, then see how you feel. If that feels doable, focus on the next step, which might be making your first few marks. If that feels okay, do the next step. But move toward doing something that might shift your energy.

○ Get out of the house. I promised I wouldn't tell you to take a long walk, but how about the micro goal of walking to the corner? And if that's okay, to the next corner. And so on. Humor me?

○ Get grounded. You'll be learning more about this later when we talk about strengthening energetic boundaries, but here's a quick tip to start. By connecting to the earth's surface, you can help your body calm down and be more balanced. Simply put your bare feet on the dirt, sand, grass, or unsealed concrete and chill out for a few minutes.

○ When chores such as doing the dishes or opening the mail feel daunting, work in small steps—aiming to open just a few envelopes in the stack of the mail or do just a few dishes.

Emotional Self-Care

○ If you feel anxious, try to move, breathe, and eat more slowly. Slowing down in this way signals to our body that we're safe to relax.

○ All of the exercises you just learned in this chapter are perfect for when you feel really freaked out, bad, or anxious. Use them in the moment as emergency tools.

Additional Ideas

○ Resist triggers. When we're in *freakout* mode, we tend to choose activities or expose ourselves to triggers that perpetuate it, perhaps because of the chaotic energy that drives it. Be gentle with yourself, and don't tune in to things or people that trigger you.

○ Reduce overwhelm. Limit social media exposure and activities, even if they are positive. Too much of a seemingly good thing can create chaos too.

○ Shift your surroundings. Your surroundings are part of the energetic relationship between you and the world. When you're stuck, you often become stuck in the midst of the patterns and energies that surround you. These micro movements in your environment can help: move the direction of your bed or furniture, change the art or colors in your room, and clean up clutter (even if you have to put it in a box to get it out of your way temporarily).

Now, let's move on to learn the main techniques we'll be using throughout this book so we can start aiming at that deeper emotional baggage we've been discussing.

3

Energy Therapy Techniques

One of the most overwhelming parts of figuring out how to feel better is figuring out *what* will help you feel better. And truth be told, I believe there are always a bunch of ways to achieve the same thing. But you have to find the way that feels best to you. This was my own biggest challenge when I first realized that talk therapy wasn't going to be the fix I wanted in terms of healing my emotional terrain. I read dozens of books and had seen so many brilliant practitioners, yet had a difficult time finding techniques that I could—and *would*—use on my own. Most of them required special tools or another person. Many required hours a day of practice. Some self-healing programs work on the premise that if you miss one session or mess up in any way at any time, you've ruined your chance of success and have to start over. And to be honest, many of them felt too "out there" or woo-woo for me.

Here's the thing we really need to focus on: using the tools is the only way they'll work. The good news is that in this chapter, you'll be learning the basics of techniques that work, don't require hours of time a day, and once you get the hang of them, will become natural for you to use anytime, anywhere. No strict rules or requirements. This will make them as easy as possible to integrate into any real-life life.

About the Techniques

As we've already touched upon, energy psychology, which is the basis of my work, is an approach that specifically addresses the relationship between the energy system and emotions, thoughts, and behavior. The energy therapy techniques in this book are all ones that specifically address emotional energy that is imbalancing or disrupting your system. By using energy therapy in this way, we know we are working with the core of who we really are—our emotional selves—to instigate true change and healing.

Our goal is for these techniques (even if not all of them) to truly become second nature to you. When this "click" happens, you're going to get the most from them. It will be hard to imagine this scenario as you first learn—similar to how on the first day of a new job we can hardly grasp that things will ever be easy, but then soon are doing the tasks of the job without thinking. This is how energy work will be for you once you get past the learning curve. I want to make sure you can use the techniques without much effort, because I know when you feel like shit, there is no extra effort to be found. But you have to stick with me through the little bumps we often hit while learning.

Each of the techniques will be used to help you release emotional energy, no matter where it's stored in your body or what symptoms it may be causing. You may remember there are various parts of the energy system, and while working with one part we are able to affect the others. Again, my techniques primarily address energy in meridians and chakras. Here is a quick lesson on meridians and chakras so you can get an idea of what they're all about. Just remember that in any system we are accessing, we are always accessing the energy body to work with emotional stress to heal down to the core.

Meridians

Meridians are energy pathways—like rivers—that flow through your entire body. Each meridian has its own name, flows along a certain pathway, is connected to a specific function in the physical body, and correlates to its own set of emotions. The triple warmer meridian, the pathway associated with the *freak out* response that you learned about earlier, is so powerful and important that I see it as its own mini energy system. Much of the work we'll be doing in this book is connected to this meridian's system.

Chakras

Chakras work differently than meridians. There are seven main chakras that run in a line up your body, each spinning at a different speed and energetic frequency. You can think of chakras as discs of energy. In fact, *chakra* is a Sanskrit word that translates to "wheel." These wheels or discs spin in different parts of the body. For instance, you have a chakra in the center of your chest (heart chakra) and one below your belly button (sacral chakra).

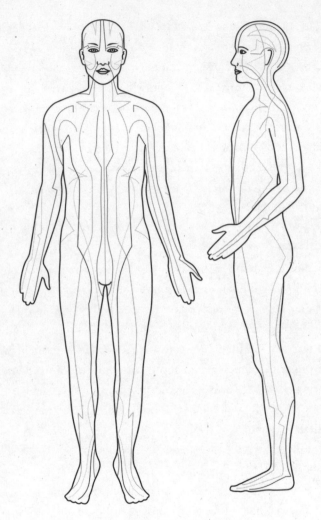

Main Meridian Channels

Chakras hold the energy of old stories, beliefs, and emotions from our lives—typically related to childhood. Like meridians, each chakra has a unique correspondence to specific locations within the body, emotions, and functions.

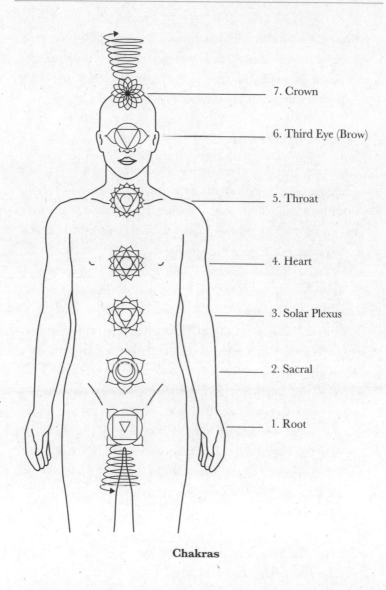

Chakras

It's through the releasing of emotional baggage and changing behaviors linked to these different parts of your energy system that we'll be pulling you out from all you've been buried by—the metaphorical *volcano*. In addition, this work will support you in creating lasting change that will help you connect to yourself—and to your sense of joy in life. The energy therapy techniques are not the cure but the catalyst to becoming your truest, best self.

Overview of Techniques

The time has come to get acquainted with the techniques you'll be using throughout the book. With the exception of the Emotional Freedom Technique (EFT), the following techniques are ones that I created myself and are now widely used around the world. As you learn the basics, you'll get a great understanding of how and why each technique works, but again, I'll be helping you apply them for the most common general blocks related to depression as we move through the next chapters.

Later in the book (part IV) you'll have an opportunity to learn how to use my techniques interchangeably and to address pretty much any emotion, belief, pattern, or stuck energy you can think of! This means you can learn to use any technique to clear a variety of emotional blocks. It can also be a very effective approach to layer techniques (use more than one) in order to clear a specific block more deeply than you might with one technique alone. You'll see examples of both of these approaches throughout the book as I guide you, and in part IV, I'll teach you how to do this for yourself too.

Here we go.

Tapping Techniques: Alternative Temple Tapping, Emotional Freedom Technique, and Chakra Tapping

Tapping describes a set of techniques used for releasing or neutralizing any emotional energy stuck in your system. Tapping allows us to mobilize blocks within the energy system by tapping certain parts of our face and body to "clear" stuck energy. Throughout your body, there are special points that can be accessed to move energy and remove blocks. Where there is an energetic imbalance, there is a corresponding block in the energy system, which contributes to emotional and physical symptoms. Gently tapping on these areas with the fingertips while we focus on how we feel or the problem at hand works to release the blocks and restore balance.

Tapping is so simple that people actually tend to overcomplicate it! You only need to focus on two things: (1) talk about the feeling or problem you have (either out loud or in your head), and (2) simultaneously tap specific points on your face or body to change the reaction to them in your energy system. That's it.

Note: If you are unable to physically tap for any reason, close your eyes and imagine this process. It may seem a little far-fetched, but because everything is energy (thoughts, emotions, and your body), it's actually surprisingly effective to go through this all in your mind. Remember, our mind and body are intricately connected. In fact, this is my favorite thing to do in the middle of the night when I can't sleep—it works without waking up my wife and helps me release my worries and fall back asleep quickly.

How Tapping Helps Us

Tapping techniques give us a way to deal with our feelings or emotional baggage in a productive way. We do this by actually bringing them up to the surface and letting go of them so we can move on. People often share with me that they are afraid to feel and deal with their feelings because they might open a Pandora's box. They worry they'll get stuck with all these "bad" feelings. But the truth is that you've already been feeling the feelings at some level (hence the depression), so the only thing you are doing now is actually dealing with and changing your reaction to them so you can stop feeling them constantly.

All of the tapping techniques you're going to learn include a "venting" process—requiring that you talk or think about the emotional stress you are wanting to release. Venting simply means saying or thinking all the things you already feel inside. If you have a hard time with this, imagine you are telling a close friend or me how you feel. Let your feelings come to the surface. None of them have to make any sense at all, but you do need to bring them up. This is key. If you are numb, that's okay. You can describe how you *think* you'd feel if you could feel anything at all.

The biggest obstacle people have to tapping that I hear is this: "I don't know what to say or think." And my answer is always, "If you have thoughts in your head, you are golden." Plus, I joke, humans *always* have something to say, opinions to voice, worries to worry about, and thoughts to express—and *now* when I'm giving you free rein, there is really *nothing* in your head? So here's the simple thing to remember: you are simply adding the action of tapping to the narration, thoughts, and feelings that you already have. It can be phrases, words, full-on complaints, disconnected thoughts, noises, or whatever comes out that expresses what you're feeling inside.

Whatever you do, don't try to be positive as you tap. You are basically tapping the bad shit *out* and using the "name it to claim it" approach so your body knows what to release. Remember, tapping is just about (1) bringing up the reality of how you feel (either out loud or in your head) and (2) tapping to let go of the energy or stress from your body. You'll be using this same process over and over, with breaks every few minutes, until you start to feel better.

At the very end of your tapping process, you'll be able to do one "round" of tapping using positive statements. This will only be for about a minute, but it feels great to end in an upbeat way.

How Tapping Works

Mechanically speaking, here's how tapping works. Imagine your dog freaks out every time the mail carrier comes to the door. Each day you tell Rufus in your most calming voice that he's okay and safe around this person, but chances are Rufus will just look at you like you don't know what you're talking about and continue to bark in fear. But if you kneel down next to him and pat him, calming him at the same time he is looking at this scary person, you'll be sending a strong signal to his body that he is safe and okay even while facing this "danger." In this scenario, you are changing how Rufus feels about this thing that is usually stressful, and ultimately you are changing the pattern of what happens to Rufus in his body when he sees the mail carrier. His system is now reprogramming itself to be okay and balanced in the presence of said person. You are not changing the circumstance but rather the reaction or stress response in the body. We're basically doing the same thing for you. We're changing what happens to you in your energy body when you are feeling difficult emotions or holding emotional baggage.

Three Tapping Techniques

There are three tapping techniques I want you to get familiar with, but don't panic, because you don't have to use them all. I only want you to be exposed to all of them so you have choices. The process for each of the techniques is based on sequentially tapping on various places on your face and body—the only difference being *where* you actually tap on your face and body.

Super easy! All these tapping techniques achieve the same thing in different ways. And they all share a very similar process, so you only have to learn one thing to gain three new tools! Let's go over each of them.

Alternate Temple Tapping (ATT): This is a technique I created that combines tapping on the temples to release emotional blocks specifically by engaging the powerful triple warmer meridian—which governs the body's *freakout* response. Because the temples are the starting point of the triple warmer meridian, I've found tapping on them to be extremely useful, especially to release the most stuck emotional energy. In this technique, we use tapping *alternately* on each side of the face with your fingertips (tap left, tap right) to activate both hemispheres of the brain. This is a process called bilateral stimulation, which is a small piece of EMDR therapy (a therapy that needs to be done with a practitioner). But the bilateral stimulation component is integrated into many types of techniques and has been shown to mediate the stress response. I find ATT to be very powerful in the "letting go" process because of how we are addressing the fight, flight, or freeze mechanism along with the emotional energy or block.

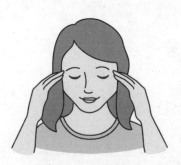

Temple Tapping Points

Emotional Freedom Technique (EFT): When I started out in my own healing, I went to a practitioner who used a specific tapping technique called Emotional Freedom Technique (EFT), developed in the 1990s by Gary Craig. EFT is a simple and effective tool based on the meridian system of energy pathways in the body. It combines the principles of acupuncture (without the needles) and talking! Studies have shown that EFT is able to rapidly reduce the emotional impact of memories and incidents that trigger emotional distress and often lead to physical pain and symptoms. Results of EFT can be shown with an electroencephalogram (EEG) machine, proving that brainwave patterns respond to the tapping. Studies have shown that after doing EFT, there are reductions in cortisol, a primary stress hormone, and these reductions are accompanied by improvements in heart rate variability, which is used to measure stress. EFT changes the reaction in the energy system, which eliminates the "charge" in the body that

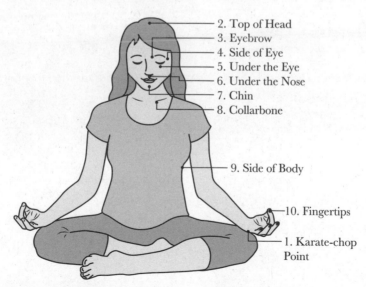

2. Top of Head
3. Eyebrow
4. Side of Eye
5. Under the Eye
6. Under the Nose
7. Chin
8. Collarbone
9. Side of Body
10. Fingertips
1. Karate-chop Point

Emotional Freedom Technique Points

accompanies that issue. However, the way I learned it was complicated, and I couldn't do it by myself. This technique is often used by practitioners and in clinical settings to address complex traumas. However, I'll be sharing the DIY version, which is simple and safe to use on your own. I've coined my way of teaching it *The Easy Amy Way!* because of the ease with which anyone can use it. I teach it to kids as young as age five and have people all over the world tell me that once they learned my version of EFT, they were finally able to get the results they'd always wanted from it.

(1) **Karate-chop point**—*Tapping point:* The outside of your hand, about halfway between the bottom of your pinky and your wrist.

(2) **Top of the head**—*Tapping point:* This is smack dab in the middle of the top of your head.

(3) **Eyebrow**—*Tapping point:* The inside corner of the eye, right where the eyebrow starts.

(4) **Side of the eye**—*Tapping point:* The outer corner of the eye, right on the bone, close to where it meets your temple.

(5) **Under the eye**—*Tapping point:* The top of the cheekbone, right under the eye.

(6) **Top lip**—*Tapping point:* This is where a mustache would be if you had one.

(7) **Chin**—*Tapping point:* In the indentation on your chin, halfway between your bottom lip and the tip of your chin.

(8) **Collarbone**—*Tapping point:* Find where you would tie a tie on your necke, then go out to the side an inch and drop directly under the collarbone.

(9) Under the arm/side of the body—*Tapping point:* This is where a bra band is, about four inches under the armpit on the side of the body.

(10) Fingertips—*Tapping point:* The lower right-hand corner of each fingernail, where it meets the cuticle. You only need to tap on the fingertips of one hand.

Chakra Tapping (CT): This technique targets a different part of the energy system than EFT. Chakra Tapping addresses energy stuck in the chakras, those spinning energy centers in the body that hold the energies of old stories and imprints from our lives. Each chakra covers a specific part of the body, correlates with specific emotions, and affects the physical area of the body where it is located. I loved studying about the chakras and, for fun, decided to apply the EFT process to them. What I found was that my emotional energies would often change more quickly or differently than they did when I used EFT. So I adapted the EFT process and call this *Chakra Tapping*, which uses the exact same format as EFT but different tapping points on the face and body.

Crown (Seventh) Chakra Tapping Point—Top of the head

Third Eye or Brow (Sixth) Chakra Tapping Point—In between the eyebrows

Throat (Fifth) Chakra Tapping Point—Front of the throat

Heart (Fourth) Chakra Tapping Point—In the middle of the chest

Solar Plexus (Third) Chakra Tapping Point—Right under the sternum at your solar plexus

Sacral (Second) Chakra Tapping Point—Just below the belly button

Root (First) Chakra Tapping Point—Top of your thighs (Pat them like you're calling a puppy up on your lap.)

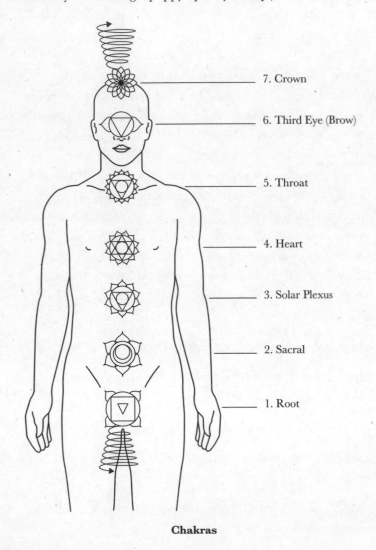

7. Crown

6. Third Eye (Brow)

5. Throat

4. Heart

3. Solar Plexus

2. Sacral

1. Root

Chakras

How to Know Which Tapping Technique to Use

I've found that using one type of tapping or another is sometimes more effective or comfortable for certain people or certain types of emotional energies. So throughout this book, when I refer to using tapping, and unless I specify a certain set of points, you are free to use whichever set of tapping points you'd like. I tend to use them interchangeably; so, like me, you may decide to use all three, depending on what you're working on. You may learn to intuitively choose whichever tapping technique works best for you at different times. And, if you aren't getting enough of a shift from one set of points, you can switch to another.

As a quick summary:

* With Alternate Temple Tapping (ATT), you are working with the fight, flight, or freeze energy dynamic.

* With Emotional Freedom Technique (EFT), you are primarily affecting the meridians.

* With Chakra Tapping (CT), you are primarily affecting the chakras.

The cool thing is that because our energy subsystems are intertwined, you are actually affecting your entire system indirectly when you use any of them. So, if you aren't getting enough of a shift from one set of points, you can switch to another. I'll make sure to remind you of all your options as we go through the process in this book.

How to Tap

I'll be walking you through these same tapping exercises in each chapter, so again, there's nothing you need to do right now except be willing to try it when it's time. If you've tried tapping before and felt clumsy, doubtful, or unsure, stick with me. I'm going to make it as easy and effective as possible for you. I'm giving you directions for the most basic version of tapping. I'm leaving out some of the "bells and whistles" that are often included because they can feel overwhelming when you're in a state of depression and just trying to get going. I'll keep things simple here for the purposes of making sure you find this technique easy enough to actually use. Again, I often get people telling me that they'd tried tapping before without results or resonance, and that my way of approaching it made all the difference for them. If you've ever been a tapping dropout like me and so many others, I want to make sure success comes easily for you this time around.

Step 1: To start, you'll focus on the emotional energy you want to release (a situation you're struggling with, conflicted about, how you feel, etc.). Examples of this can be "feeling sad," "worrying about my dad," or "afraid I'll never feel better."

Step 2: We always start by tapping on the *karate-chop point* on the outside edge of the hand—think of how someone performing

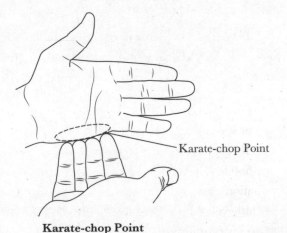

Karate-chop Point

Karate-chop Point

karate might "chop" at a block or other person. We do this for the purpose of releasing what's called in therapeutic terminology a *psychological reversal,* which means having a subconscious resistance to letting go of the problem you are experiencing. You learned about this phenomenon already in the previous chapter. Along with tapping on the karate-chop point, we use a certain formulaic statement that acknowledges to the body that you have a particular issue but also sends a message that you can release it and move on to heal. We will say this phrase three times in a row as we tap continuously:

Even though I have this _____ (describe the problem you are releasing, briefly), *I choose to let it go.*

Note: Alternatively, you can substitute "I choose to let it go" with "I can be okay anyway." I typically use one of these two phrases—or both!—whenever I do tapping of any kind. But you can use any positive affirmation you wish.

Step 3: Next, you'll start tapping on the set of points that corresponds to whichever technique you are using—Alternate Temple Tapping, Chakra Tapping, or Emotional Freedom Technique. As you cycle through the rest of the points that come after the karate-chop point, you will be "venting" (out loud or in your head) about how you're feeling or the problem you're experiencing. You can imagine telling someone close to you if it helps the process. You'll keep tapping for several minutes, taking breaks as you need for a few deep breaths. As you tap, you're going to continue using the "venting" method to talk about the emotional energy (emotions, thoughts, sensations, and feelings) you want to release. Remember, it can be anything you think or feel about it. No one else will ever know what you say or think.

For Emotional Freedom Technique (EFT) and Chakra Tapping (CT), you'll tap about 5–7 times on each point (but no need to count or be exact). You can use just one hand to do this. For EFT, you can tap the points on just one side of the face and body. For Alternate Temple Tapping (ATT), you'll tap alternately and continuously on your temples (for example, you tap your right temple with three or four fingertips on your right hand, then tap left with three or four fingertips of your left hand, and so on). This will quickly form a nice rhythm once you get started. As a reminder, here are the tapping points for each of the three techniques. Remember, you only need to choose one to work with.

Temple Tapping Points: At your temples on each side. If you only have the physical use of one hand, you can use that hand to tap the temples alternately.

Emotional Freedom Technique Points: Top of the head—*Tapping point:* This is smack dab in the middle of the top of your head. Eyebrow—*Tapping point:* The inside corner of the eye, right where the eyebrow starts. Side of the eye—*Tapping point:* The outer corner of the eye, right on the bone, close to where it meets your temple. Under the eye—*Tapping point:* The top of the cheekbone, right under the eye. Top lip—*Tapping point:* This is where a mustache would be if you had one. Chin—*Tapping point:* In the indentation on your chin, halfway between your bottom lip and the tip of your chin. Collarbone—*Tapping point:* Find where you would tie a tie on your neck, then go out to the side an inch and drop directly under the collarbone. Under the arm/side of the body—*Tapping point:* This is where a bra band is, about four inches under the armpit on the side of the body. Fingertips—*Tapping point:* The lower right-hand corner of each fingernail, where it meets the cuticle. You only need to tap on the fingertips of one hand.

Chakra Tapping Points: Crown (Seventh) Chakra—*Tapping Point:* Top of the head. Third Eye or Brow (Sixth) Chakra—*Tapping Point:* In between the eyebrows. Throat (Fifth) Chakra—*Tapping Point:* Front of the throat. Heart (Fourth) Chakra—*Tapping Point:* In the middle of the chest. Solar Plexus (Third) Chakra—*Tapping Point:* Right under the sternum at your solar plexus. Sacral (Second) Chakra—*Tapping Point:* Just below the belly button. Root (First) Chakra—*Tapping Point:* Top of your thighs (pat them like you're calling a puppy up on your lap).

Step 4: When you're ready to wrap up your tapping, regardless of which tapping technique you've used, you'll tap on all the points for about another minute (which I refer to as another "round" throughout the tapping scripts in this book), repeating "I can be okay now" or another positive affirmation to help you end on a positive note. But you'll only do this at the very end. You are not using tapping effectively if you are trying to tap on the positive *unless* you've worked on releasing the yucky stuff first.

How Long to Tap For

This is a question I get all the time, and it's so hard to answer. I usually start with about ten minutes of tapping and see how I feel (but if you only have five minutes of time, that's okay too). Once you are done, you'll want to check in with how you feel. If you feel like you need more releasing (which you very likely will), repeat the four steps until you start to feel a positive shift.

You are essentially tapping with the goal of feeling better, but obviously this may not happen right away. In fact, I often have a delayed reaction where I don't feel much better until hours later, or even a few days later. You will have to find your own flow with tapping and how long you do it.

As a guideline, it's not uncommon at all to have to work on something over several sessions to start feeling better. So make sure you stick with it and just keep going. It's almost guaranteed that one or two rounds won't be enough (although you may get lucky and feel so much better very quickly).

Thymus Test and Tap (TTT) Technique

Thymus Test and Tap also utilizes tapping, but I did not include it in the tapping techniques above because it works in a completely different way and encompasses much more than tapping alone. Thymus Test and Tap is used to release individual emotions lodged in the body that we may not be aware of. It's a simple technique that works in two parts: first, by identifying the stuck emotions in the body, even if you don't know what or where they are; and second, by utilizing the powerhouse that is your thymus gland to release those emotions and rebalance your energy system for full integration.

Many natural and integrative practitioners use intuitive testing, or applied kinesiology (a technique used to detect weaknesses in the body, which you'll be learning in part IV), to identify "stressors" negatively affecting a patient or to determine beneficial remedies to help a patient. They do this by using vials or lists of different substances and observing the body's reaction in relationship to them. Integrative nutritionists often use food frequency lists or vials along with testing to discover which foods or substances someone may be having negative reactions to. Integrative practitioners and homeopaths often use lists of microbes to help detect parasites, viruses, or bacteria harming their patients. Some practitioners, like myself, use lists of emotions, affirmations, and beliefs to identify the emotional blocks the patient is dealing with. In this same way, we'll be using a list of emotions that I created, based on years of experience, to identify emotions causing stress in your body so that we know exactly what you need to release to feel better.

The key to the effectiveness of this technique does not have anything to do with my specific list of emotions; it's the combination of finally identifying what's been stuck inside of you along with engaging the thymus gland—the central gland of the body's immune system—to release that emotional energy and expedite healing.

Your thymus gland is responsible for making T cells to help protect you against allergies, autoimmune diseases, and immunodeficiency. It's located in the upper part of the chest, behind the breastbone. The thymus is close to your heart and is sometimes called "the heart's protector." The heart is, of course, the seat of our emotional center. In terms of the energy system, the thymus gland regulates the energy flow throughout your entire body. It is almost immediately impacted when we experience emotional stress. Because the thymus gland is connected to the rest of the body's energy system, it has great power in emotional healing. By tapping the thymus gland in a specific way, you can release emotions stuck in any part of your system. The percussive effect of the specific tapping in this place sends a force of energy through your thymus gland to clear the emotional block or imbalance wherever it is in your system. You don't need to know where it is. As you tap, you are also rebalancing and strengthening the thymus gland, allowing it to recalibrate.

Each person can have thousands of emotions stuck in their bodies (this is totally normal!), but you don't need to clear even close to that amount to start feeling better (or ever, actually). Using the TTT technique can often result in immediate improvement, but working with it should be seen as a marathon and not a sprint. I typically release up to twenty or so emotions at once, but it doesn't stop there. I continuously come back to this technique to do more and more. In this way, even if we have lots of emotions stuck in the body, we can clear enough to make a "dent" in the mountain of them, which can have a great positive impact on how we feel.

How Thymus Test and Tap Helps Us

While tapping using ATT, EFT, or CT allows us to use our own language and descriptions of our challenges, TTT gives us the ability to target and clear specific individual emotions—such as guilt, resentment, or fear—that are stuck in our body, even if we have no idea what they are. These emotions may have originated many years ago but are still affecting you greatly today. Or they may be newer emotions that you have not yet consciously identified in terms of how you feel (we get used to saying "I'm depressed" or "I'm anxious" and sometimes lose the ability to discern what the real emotions beneath these statements are).

This is a more mechanical way to find and release emotions, which can be beneficial when we feel bad but really can't connect with why. With TTT, we are simply identifying an emotion and releasing it, identifying another and releasing it, and so on. This process is very powerful as another great way to access emotional energy stored in our bodies; however, I shy away from using this technique solely because it doesn't require any self-introspection or recognition of patterns, which I believe is absolutely necessary to make sure we don't re-create all that we're releasing.

Because this technique was created to utilize the powerful role of the thymus gland and the energy system, it has a very special MO. When we use Thymus Test and Tap, we are getting a *triple affect* by affecting the immune system, nervous system, and heart field energy all at once.

How to Do Thymus Test and Tap

To release emotions in our system that are unknown to us, we first need to identify what they are. What I mean by this is that we need to know exactly which emotions you've been carrying around before we can use the thymus tapping process to release them. Even a single emotional energy that is cleared can free up a huge amount of energy in your system or make a dent in that mountain of emotions causing you to feel so depressed. So don't underestimate the power of each release.

Take a look at this list of emotions we'll be using. I've left some blank spaces so that you can add any you think of on your own.

Note: On every other emotion list I've seen, the word "anxiety" is included. I consider anxiety more of a description (feeling "anxious") than a true feeling. What we tend to describe as "anxiety" is typically another suppressed emotion, or emotions, trying to bubble up. This, undoubtedly, makes us feel anxious. However, in an effort to really get to the bottom of anxiety, I have omitted it so that you can learn to dig deeper and address the true emotions. Any single emotion on this chart could cause "anxiety" if it were suppressed. Therefore, releasing any emotion on this chart could also help alleviate it. The same goes for the feeling of "depression."

Step 1: Identify an emotion to work with. You may be wondering how in the world we'll figure out which emotions need to be released. Luckily, our bodies are wise far beyond what we are aware of. There is a part of you that already knows which emotions are stuck and where they are. Here are two very easy and effective ways to pull into your awareness the emotions that are contributing to depression.

THYMUS TEST AND TAP (TTT) UNPROCESSED EMOTIONS	
Section 1	*Section 2*
Abandoned	Helpless
Fearful	Hopeless
Grief-stricken	Heavy
Unloved	Impatient
Intimidated	Out of control
Criticized	Defensive
Judged	Frustrated
Hated	Panicked
Berated	Insecure
Worthless	Powerless
Attacked	Shocked
Betrayed	Failure
Disconnected	Stressed
Section 3	*Section 4*
Rejected	Vulnerable
Angry	Unsupported
Guilty	Undeserving
Resentful	Ashamed
Blamed	Overwhelmed
Indecisiveness	Bullied
Disgusted	Lonely
Conflicted	Alone
Confused	Regretful
Nervous	Disappointed
Unsafe	Discarded
Worried	Excluded
Hurt	Desperate
Resistant	Traumatized

Use the finger swirl method. Sit quietly and ask yourself what emotion in your body might be trying to get your attention. We're going to use a process to let your body intuitively guide you. Close your eyes and very gently swirl your pointer finger all over the list of emotions. You can make big circles or any shape you want, but try to cover the entire list. When you feel called to stop, stop while holding your finger in place. What's happening is that your body is actually picking up on the emotion you need to release. It may seem like you're being very random, but this is actually quite an accurate way to do this.

Alternatively, use muscle testing. In part IV of this book (chapter 10), I teach you how to use applied kinesiology, often called *muscle testing*, to identify specific emotional energies stuck in your body. This is a great way of communicating with the subconscious mind for answers and information. As I said, we'll get to that later—but I want you to know where it is in case you'd like to peek ahead.

Step 2: Tap your thymus seven times repetitively to release. Now that you have identified the feeling that's stuck in your body, you are ready to tap your thymus to clear or neutralize it. You will release the first emotion, and then repeat the process as many times as you want to release additional emotions. Once you get the hang of this, you'll be doing it very quickly and, if you're anything like myself and my clients, even squeezing it into your five-minute tea or pee breaks during the day.

Simply tap at least seven times firmly over your thymus gland with the fingertips of one hand. If you want to tap more times, that's fine, but seven is the average that I discovered works for most people across the board. You'll often start to release the emotion on the second or third tap, but keep going just to be complete. I know a few people who can "feel" when the emotion releases, so they use their intuition and just tap until that happens, even if it's many more times than seven. Many people yawn as a signal the emotion is released—myself included—but it doesn't happen to me every single time, and it doesn't happen to every person. Just trust that you are releasing, even if you don't get any sure signal from your body.

Your thymus gland is about an inch below the notch of your neck, where a bowtie would sit. The gland itself is behind your breastbone, so you won't be able to see or feel it. However, tapping on the chest over it will do the trick because of the reverberation of tapping. I like to use the mantra *Releasing, releasing, releasing* or *Let go, let go, let go* as I tap. Because you are likely very much in the pattern of "holding on," this verbal cue (even if repeated in your head) is very powerful in retraining your body to "let go"—an important part of healing depression.

Whenever we use this technique, I'll be guiding you to identify which specific emotions are stuck in your body.

Step 3: Begin again at Step 1 and repeat as many times as needed. Again, each person has so many emotions that I want to remind you that using this technique for any challenge we address in this book isn't a one-time process. I bet I've done hundreds of sessions on myself using this technique alone. The great part is that you'll probably be pretty excited to do them since this process is so easy and effective.

Note: This technique can be used to release emotions related to very specific parameters, such as a person, or a part of your body that is experiencing symptoms. You'll learn more about how to explore in this way in part IV.

The Sweep Technique

The Sweep technique is a script that you repeat in order to clear subconscious blocks and beliefs. No tapping required! I created The Sweep as a way to "sweep" blocks out of the subconscious mind. The Sweep works by working *with* the subconscious mind (the only way it'll cooperate) and offering it the freedom to let go of what no longer serves us. I wrote The Sweep with very particular wording that proved, over all of my testing, to be extremely powerful where other techniques were not. Using The Sweep's gentle conversational script, we actually guide the subconscious mind to choose freedom from harmful beliefs or blocks that have been keeping us stuck. The Sweep can be done by simply reading the script out loud, or in your head, or recording it for yourself on your phone so you can listen back and repeat it.

How The Sweep Helps Us

The Sweep's magic is found in harnessing the conscious-subconscious mind partnership that's necessary for healing. The technique lets us reprogram the subconscious mind in a simple, nonthreatening way. The Sweep is *not* hypnotherapy, but it has a similarity in that it relaxes the body and brain in a way that allows us to change old and stubborn programming without constant resistance. A lot of people zone out as they use this technique, losing their place in the script or suddenly forgetting what they were saying. If you record it on your phone and then listen to it instead of reading it, and if you are like me, you might even fall asleep! This is actually completely normal. You will be aware and in total control. It's just very, very relaxing.

The Sweep's power comes in the form of fulfilling what we need in order to change at a core level. It lets us acknowledge that we have this issue and that we choose to release it. The Sweep allows us to engage our conscious mind by repeating the powerful phrases that give us permission and direction to heal, and it subtly encourages our subconscious mind to feel safe enough to release the old, outdated programming and choose healthier programming. The verbiage is so kind and gentle that it helps us trust the process at every level, being interpreted by the subconscious mind as a friend rather than a foe. Because change happens when the subconscious and conscious minds work together, this technique is going to be the easiest game changer ever.

How to Do The Sweep

The only thing you need to do during The Sweep is personalize it to target exactly what you are trying to release. There are two fill-in-the-blank spaces within the script. In the first blank, you'll simply plug in what you want to release or let go of. In the second blank, which is at the end of the script, you plug in what you want to install (a direction for healthier programming). I will be leading you through this process during our time together, but I created The Sweep script with a very specific approach in mind to make it fail-proof. Because the subconscious mind can resist change if forced, I start with the phrase *I am now free* for almost every sentence of The Sweep script. Freedom is a natural human desire, and it is counterintuitive to resist it—even for the stubborn subconscious mind.

Finally, we replace, or install, a new and more positive direction that will support our well-being. This will take the place of what we let go of, ensuring there is no feeling of "void," which can happen even when we release or lose something that's not healthy for us. You can choose any beneficial installation here: a positive emotion, a healthy belief, a new energy (such as "the energy of joy"), and so on. You may need to repeat The Sweep several times to completely release the energy.

In chapter 10, where you'll learn muscle testing, I'll show you how you can determine beforehand how many times to read The Sweep script (and then how to check afterward to make sure it was effective). But for now, I suggest you read it three times as a start. Don't be concerned, though, if you need to do it many more times to feel a shift. Even eight to ten isn't unheard of. You do not need to do them all in a row, though.

The Sweep Script

Even though I have this _____ (describe what you want to release), I acknowledge it's no longer working for me.

I give my subconscious full permission to help me clear it, from all of my cells in all of my body, permanently and completely.

I am now free to thank it for serving me in the past.

I am now free to release all resistances to letting it go.

I am now free to release all ideas that I need this in order to stay safe.

I am now free to release all ideas that I need it for any reason.

I am now free to release all feelings that I don't deserve to release it.

I am now free to release all conscious and subconscious causes for this energy.

I am now free to release all conscious and subconscious reasons for holding on to it.

I am now free to release all harmful patterns, emotions, and memories connected to it.

I am now free to release all generational or past-life energies keeping it stuck.

All of my being is healing and clearing this energy now, including any stress response stored in my cells.

Healing, healing, healing.

Clearing, clearing, clearing.

It is now time to install _____ (insert a new, healthy energy such as "the energy of moving forward," "the feeling of being content," or "the belief that I can feel better now").

Installing, installing, installing. Installing, installing, installing. And so it is done.

Finishing Each Energy Therapy Session: Install Positive Emotions

After I do an energy work session, whether it's five minutes or forty-five minutes, and no matter what techniques I use, I like to do a quick wrap-up by "installing" positive emotions. To do this, you can use the approach you learned for Thymus Test and Tap. While it's always good to release the old, yucky stuff, I find that giving your body a healthier replacement tends to support the complete integration and healing process. I don't think there's any danger in skipping it, but after you've carried something around for so long, we don't want your body to sense an emptiness once you release it and feel any need to find or re-create something nonbeneficial again.

To install positive emotions, you'll use the following positive emotion list to identify each emotion in the same way you did earlier, and then simply tap seven times firmly over your thymus gland. As you do this, hold the intention of tapping this energy *into* your body. I typically install three positive emotions, but you can do as many as you'd like.

THYMUS TEST AND TAP (TTT) POSITIVE EMOTIONS	
Section 1	*Section 2*
Able	Comforted
Abundant	Connected
Accepting	Content
Accepted	Decisive
Adaptable	Empowered
Appreciated	Encouraged
Assertive	Energetic
Reassured	Flowing
At ease	Forgiven
Brave	Free
Inspired	Grounded
Joyful	Happy
Light	Deserving
Protected	Loved
Section 3	*Section 4*
Secure	Trusting
Soothed	Valued
Strong	Willing
Supported	Calm
Grateful	Centered
Important	Confident
Included	Healed
Independent	Hopeful
Acknowledged	Open
Relaxed	Optimistic
Empowered	Peaceful
Understood	Positive

Processing and Improvement Time

Often, there is a delay from when you use the techniques to when the energy clears from your body completely. Because our energy field extends beyond our body, the energy you are clearing from your system may process out of your field slowly. When you learn muscle testing, you can use it to check your work and make sure you've cleared energy completely. However, it's important to keep in mind that the results of the work may not be immediate. The reason for this is that it takes time for the body to come back into balance once you release the obstacles or blocks. As an analogy, you may put a healing salve on your skin directly after a sunburn, but the effect is not immediate. The salve is a remedy to support the skin, but then the skin must do the healing work.

This applies to our work too. First, you must give the body the support it needs to heal (in our case, releasing emotional baggage)—and then the body must do the work of healing. So there is often a lag time in you doing the work and starting to feel better. Not always, but that is definitely the norm. It really can take time. Just keep chipping away and know the healing is happening.

Next comes the part you've been waiting for: the healing work. You now officially know everything you need to know to *start*, which is truly the hardest part. But we're going to do it all together. It's time. We are going to be actively healing the energetic root of the problem, carefully choosing exercises that will help us *un*do in order to actually affect change—and, most importantly, reconnect to the lightest, real-deal happiest version of ourselves.

PART II

Heal Yourself:

Going In to Get You Out
Releasing Emotional Baggage

We often think of stress as our day-to-day and bigger life challenges. But stress is in fact mostly happening inside us. To heal depression, we must identify and release the stress that is keeping us buried—our emotions, traumas, and beliefs that no longer serve us.

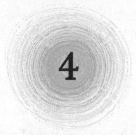

4

Clear Harmful Beliefs

Beliefs are a framework for how we take in the world. They are essentially commands from the brain about how to perceive reality: based on your past experiences, recognized patterns, other people's messages about us, knowledge we've gathered, interpretations (meanings we've made), and environment. Our brain then directs its behavior based on our beliefs.

While there are many theories about belief formation and function from philosophers to neuroscientists, there is little debate about just how much of our lives are affected by what we believe. In fact, much of your current life, how you relate to the world, what you see, and what you think—the good and the bad—has been built, perhaps frighteningly, upon what you think you think.

In other words, how you see the world is aligned to what you *already* believe to be true. Beliefs are yet another way we try to feel safe. Beliefs are a way to quickly make sense of events in life; they help us predict what might happen in the future so we can protect ourselves. But what if those beliefs are blocking us from health? Happiness? And more?

In this chapter you'll learn what beliefs are, how they are affecting you, and how you can change them to change the way you see and experience your entire life.

What Beliefs Are

Beliefs are not fact, even though they may feel like it. A belief is simply an idea you perceive, or believe, to be true. Beliefs that are positive, such as "I matter" or "I can heal," act as positive affirmations in your life, helping you to feel good and move forward. But it's very common to have beliefs that are harmful to you, meaning you bought into an idea that is working against you. Examples of these beliefs would be "I don't matter" and "I'm unable to heal." You can think of these types of beliefs as negative affirmations, in which we affirm something undesirable (or unhealthy) over and over. This creates a negative impact on your life.

Beliefs are the equivalent of *meanings* we make in our lives—the takeaway messages we are left with after computing information from our life's experiences. And our messages about life pretty much rule our world. That's why beliefs are one of the largest contributors to depression and one of the greatest impediments to overcoming it.

What makes this scarier is the suggestion that these beliefs of ours are typically formed by the age of seven. We already know that our genes are not the major controlling factor of our biology, as we once thought they were. Instead, our biology is greatly influenced by signals and programming that comes from outside of us. The dominant frequencies of the brain from birth until age seven are *delta* and *theta*—the same state achieved during hypnosis. In other words, delta and theta operate below the level of consciousness or awareness. This means that children up to age seven are basically living in a trance-like state, open to programming of perceptions, experiences, and more. At this early age, we lack the critical thinking or filtering ability to control or make sense of what to download. This is how and when our primary perspective of the world gets programmed. Because the primitive brain tends to prioritize efficiency, once we are programmed, it's our tendency to resist changing its programming, even if it makes no sense for our lives anymore.

All of this means that, even as adults, we are living by much of the programming that occurred before we hit double-digit ages. Oh boy. It's no wonder much of our thinking is stressing us out. We are essentially living by a very outdated playbook that we got at a young age.

While this sounds, well, depressing, it's not all that bad (at least, not now that you're privy to this information). Releasing these limiting or harmful beliefs is one of the most life-changing practices I've used for myself and with clients. I liken transforming beliefs to unsubscribing from email accounts that send you spam and use tricky marketing tactics to make you believe in a product. In a similar process, we can stop receiving these bullshit messages from our brain in order to move on with our lives.

Now that you understand what beliefs are, let me show you exactly how we can change our lives if we work with them.

Why What We Believe Is So Important

The mind is the intermediary between our beliefs and reality. All cells come from the same source, but it's the programming of them that influences our beliefs and behavior. Here's a recap of how it works. Your mind is designed to "drive" your life according to your programming. Your programming is then used to create or direct your thoughts and behaviors, which are then reflected as your reality.

This concept makes perfect sense when you think in the context of different cultures. Imagine two children, one being raised in India and the other in Australia. The structures of the cells within each child are the same, but the programming from culture and environment is what makes up how each of them sees the world.

Let's take a look at the breakdown of how beliefs work to really get a picture of how they affect our entire lives.

* Based primarily on our early childhood experiences, our subconscious mind perceives certain messages or takeaways that form the way we see ourselves and the world (our beliefs).

* The subconscious creates rules or directions to attach to each belief, based on the past. For example, *this* is good or *this* is bad, or when *this* happens then *this* other thing happens.

* These beliefs created a tainted lens, which we see everything through, dictating our lives and influencing our decisions, behavior, and feelings.

* Our perceptions become reinforced by our skewed perspectives and beliefs, which enforce neural pathways in the brain (circuitry that controls our habits, thoughts, and behaviors).

You can now imagine how problematic it is when our programming is stressful, inaccurate, and limiting. We count on our programming to be in line with what we desire for our lives. But our programming came from our parents' programming, society's programming, and our own meanings we made—often during times of emotional stress. This is especially troublesome because trauma and overwhelm make it difficult to take in new or accurate information.

In the 1990s, Daniel T. Gilbert, a psychology researcher at the University of Texas at Austin, conducted a fascinating study with two of his colleagues. Subjects were asked to read two crime reports, each containing both deliberately true and false information. Researchers color-coded the true and false statements, making it clear to the subjects which was which. Some of the subjects were interrupted or distracted (aka overwhelmed or stressed) as they were given the false information about the defendant. Results of the study concluded that all the interrupted subjects believed the false information was *true*, even though it was clearly marked as false.

This gives us such important insight into how our own negative beliefs are formed. Unfortunately, because negative beliefs are typically formed in the midst of trauma or emotionally stressful experiences, where we make meanings quickly in an effort to cope and move on, you can see why we might not get it all right, huh? This means that perceptions made under pressure are likely to be embraced as truth, even when we gain better or more accurate information or realizations later on.

Imagine that as a young child, you were afraid to speak up in your house. Or maybe this is true and you don't have to imagine. Maybe it's because you have a parent who discouraged communication about difficult emotions because they themselves weren't emotionally healthy, or maybe it's because you were a sensitive kid and were afraid to share your feelings. Let's say that one evening, you were really upset by something your brother had said to you before you left for school. When you finally mustered the courage to bring it up to your mom, she brushed it off and told you to stop being so dramatic. In the midst of trying so hard to voice your feelings to her, and in her dismissing you, you perceive that you don't matter. You take this in as the truth and run with it for your whole life. Perhaps this and other meanings you made have been discussed in therapy. Yet even with corrected information and the understanding that your mom may have been simply having a bad day or acting from her own place of discomfort with emotions, you continue believing this belief. That's because the perception was programmed. And because you believe it, you tend to perceive it in all areas of your life—when your boss doesn't have time to talk to you, when a friend cancels your coffee date, when your spouse forgets to do the chores. As you see more examples of "I don't matter," the belief gets practiced, further validating what you believe.

Clinging to old beliefs is just another way we cling to safety when we're overwhelmed or stressed. It feels "safe" because it's familiar programming. And it feels dangerous to challenge it, because of the *do not move* rule that comes into play when we're suspended in *freakout* mode. But living by these old beliefs is anything but safe.

Remember that the subconscious controls 95 percent of our lives; so, by accessing and transforming beliefs, we can literally redirect our realties. That's why it's so important to work toward changing beliefs. Essentially, anything you believe that is adding stress to or limiting your life needs to be addressed.

The problem is that we can't convince or pressure ourselves into a new way of seeing things. We need to change the subconscious programming of your beliefs, which we'll be doing together in this chapter.

Types of Beliefs

There are two main types of beliefs that could be affecting you, each in different ways: beliefs that *contribute* to depression, and beliefs that *block* you from overcoming it. In each of these cases, you are believing something that directly contradicts the goal you have of feeling good. But almost all beliefs have a singular common thread of creating a feeling that you are unsafe in the world (emotionally or physically). In fact, "I am unsafe" is, in and of itself, one of the most common beliefs I see. This belief tends to direct behavior such as shying away from social interactions, feeling fearful about life in general, and having unfulfilling intimate relationships.

Let's look deeper at the types of beliefs to help you really grasp the importance of this topic. You aren't going to need to categorize your own beliefs in any way, so I'm sharing the types just for your own understanding—no need to remember the different types or how they work. The other good news is that we address both types the very same way, so this will be easy.

Beliefs That Contribute to Depression

The first type of belief acts as a pair of negativity goggles. These types of beliefs essentially created bad feelings by making us view ourselves and the world in a largely negative way. These beliefs can occur because other people told us negative things about our environment or ourselves, or we perceived them ourselves (by making meanings from our own experiences). Examples of beliefs of this nature are "I'm worthless," "The world is dangerous," and "I have no power over my life." This type of belief disconnects you from your inner being by causing pain, fear, and insecurity. Basically, these beliefs give you a negative perspective of yourself and the world. They are tricky because we tend to dig our heels in about them and argue that some of them really are true. But you have to be very careful here that your brain isn't tricking you based on its own set of programmed "rules." Let's go over an example of this type of belief.

Imagine you are five years old and tell your parents that you hate your new baby sibling and get punished or reprimanded for it. This is a common thing for kids to say, which is why I use this example, but parents can sometimes be really reactive to this, understandably. Now, let's suppose your sibling gets badly hurt shortly after this incident where you stated you hated him or her. Your takeaway from that experience could be that the "bad thing" you said caused something bad to happen—which then creates the belief "I can't make mistakes." This belief can not only contribute to depression but also lend itself to the deeply held pattern of perfectionism, in which you might believe doing everything right would prevent something else like this from ever happening again.

Beliefs That Block You from Healing

The next type of belief actually makes it difficult to overcome depression and stops you from feeling good. These beliefs make you believe you *need* or *deserve* to feel like shit. Even as you are doing everything to feel better, your subconscious mind has programming to make you believe you can't, or shouldn't, feel good for some reason. The bottom line with these beliefs is that your subconscious mind believes you are better off stuck where you are now than feeling better.

This belief is linked to subconscious conflict (or sabotage) that keeps you from getting better. I see this across the board with my clients and students. And for me, this was the type of belief that I feel stalled my own healing the most. You already know a lot about resistance from being in *freakout* mode. Beliefs are the very powerful way that same dynamic plays out in the subconscious mind. Beliefs result in a part of you (conscious) that wants to get better and another part of you (subconscious) that is resisting it because it believes you shouldn't or can't.

Using the example of the baby sibling again, let's look at this second type of belief as it relates to that story. Because of how you might have perceived your mistake as tied to your sibling's injury, your takeaway might be that you *deserved to be punished*. This could easily become a rule you live by, which causes you to feel like you deserve to feel bad—to be depressed. This could create a situation where your belief that you deserve punishment directly contradicts your wanting to feel good and find happiness in life. But because your subconscious programming is so ingrained, it would likely be winning for a long time (before our work together, of course).

The most common way I see this type of belief show up is with a person believing at a deep level that they are safer or better off in some way stuck at home, depressed, than they are out in a world that feels overwhelming in some way. This has been absolutely true for me in the past. When life became too much and I didn't know how to deal with my emotions, get out of a toxic relationship, and be honest about my career desires, I think I subconsciously took myself "out of the game" with illness. Of course, there were other factors, but this one was major for me. So big, in fact, that working from this standpoint created a huge positive shift in my health even when nothing else had worked.

In both of the scenarios we just went over, subconscious programming was driving the train. You might be overwhelmed thinking about all the harmful beliefs you could have, but don't worry. You don't have to reprogram them all in order to see improvement. And it's actually quite easy to change them. Phew.

Tips for Thinking about Beliefs

Before I ask you to think back on your life so we can figure out what's keeping you stuck, I want to say one important thing. It's essential not to get caught up in feeling bad about all the seemingly "crazy" (I use this word lovingly and lightly) beliefs you might discover. Having beliefs is part of being human. In fact, when I teach my workshops and online classes, I often joke that we're all just going to agree to feel a little crazy together and pretend like it's totally normal (which actually, it is). Our goal here isn't to start figuring out who screwed us up and how, either. What we want to do is identify undesirable beliefs, especially from childhood, and reprogram you into an adult who believes *good* things that will help you feel better. Because unless you are totally fine with the seven-year-old version of yourself calling the shots for your life, it's time to audit and update those mental records of yours.

Later in this chapter I'll give you an extensive list of very common beliefs associated with depression, but I really want you to learn how to identify them on your own too. The ones you come up with first will likely be the ones that you are most driven by. Another reason it's great to know how to identify your own beliefs is because if a challenge comes up for you in the future, you'll be able to quickly figure out if some of what you're believing is contributing to it.

Here we go. You may want to use your notebook to make notes as far as what resonates for you as you read.

Listen to Your Mental Commentary

Many of our thoughts are simply things we believe. This makes listening to our own inner narration one of the best ways to figure out what we believe—and if believing it is a good thing. For example, do you hear your mental commentary reveal things like "I always mess up," "No one appreciates me," or "Life is always a struggle"? All of these examples are *beliefs*. While they may seem like fact, they are just a narration of how you perceive life, picked up from your childhood or assumptions. Telling them apart can be a bit tricky at first, but it can help to ask yourself this question: "Do I know 100 percent this is true in all circumstances and could be proven as fact?" If you answer yes, I'll let you assume it's true. But if not, it's most likely what you've come to believe.

Observe How You Feel

Often, we feel a certain way because of a belief triggering those feelings. Do you feel sad because your friends didn't include you in an outing? Could there be a belief or message you are taking away from that? Perhaps the belief "I am an outcast" fits for you in this scenario. How about a situation where you are having a hard time finding a job? Is there a belief you have that skews your perception of the entire job search? What about the belief "I'll never get a job"? See if you can dig for an underlying "message" in your feelings at any given time. By doing this, you'll be cherry-picking the "belief" that might be attached.

Identify Your Takeaway Message

Because beliefs are learned, asking some questions about what you believe can be an easy and enlightening way to discover which beliefs are holding you back. Basically, we're looking for what messages you've learned about each topic. What have you been taught? What is your "takeaway" idea about it? Sometimes, thinking in terms of our parents' "advice" on each topic helps because we often learn beliefs from our family unit. For instance, if your parents said, "Money doesn't grow on trees," you likely took away the message "There's not/never enough money" or "I need to worry for when there's no more." You can probably recognize how either of these beliefs could drive money fears or insecurities in your life. Repeating the mantra "There's never enough," even at a subconscious level, can be very damaging. Simply translating what you learned about something will give you a jackpot of beliefs.

Identify Your Beliefs

To start this process, I want you to make a list in your notebook of all the beliefs you may have in each of the categories or themes that follow. Feel free to refer back to the tips I just offered as you go through each category. Remember, to identify your beliefs, simply think in terms of "messages" you have about each category. If some positive beliefs come up, yay! You don't need to write them down because we want to leave those just as they are—but it's always nice to notice them.

It's okay if you find out you have contradictory beliefs. This is very normal. For instance, "I'm unable to get well" and "I can only get well if I have more money" can't both be true; and in this case, neither are actually fact.

If you simply look at *what areas* of life you're struggling with, you'll be surprised how many beliefs are there to discover. I guarantee that where you struggle most is where there are the most beliefs behind the struggle. In fact, "I need to struggle" is a belief of its own, which we will be clearing together at the end of this chapter.

Beliefs about Self-Esteem

Self-esteem relates to how you feel about yourself. Beliefs in this category will be things you believe related to who you are, how you relate to the world, and your opinions and judgments of yourself. Questions to ask yourself here are, *What do I think about myself?*

What do I believe is true about me? How have other people's perceptions influenced what I believe about myself?

Here are some common examples: "I'm stupid," "I'm not a good daughter," "I'm too slow at things," "There is nothing good about me," "I'm not good enough," "I don't have what it takes to succeed/be happy," "I don't deserve to feel good," "I'm unlovable," "I'm 'too much,'" "I'm difficult," "I have to try harder than everyone else," "No one cares about me," "I don't matter."

Beliefs about Career

This category relates to your work life. This is important to pay attention to even if you feel you don't have a career, or don't currently work, as you'll likely find beliefs to work with there anyway.

Examples: "I'm so behind in life/work," "I'm worthless because I don't have a career," "My job is going to kill me," "I'll never be able to do what I love," "Work has to be miserable," "If I'm happy at work then I'm not working hard enough," "I need to be stressed to prove I care."

Beliefs about Health

Your health is anything that relates to the well-being of your mind and body. These beliefs are typically where we end up subconsciously sabotaging our health. I was a pro at this. I believed so many false messages that they were running my health more than my actual body was!

Examples: "I'm unable to heal," "No one can help me," "I'll be like this forever," "If I don't eat perfectly I'll get sick," "My body is weak," "I can only heal if _____," "It's not worth all the work," "Feeling bad is just my fate," "I deserve to be sick," "I'll always be sick because it's in my genes," "Other people can get better but I can't."

The biggest blocks in terms of beliefs I see with clients in this category are related to why part of them (the subconscious mind) believes they *need* depression, anxiety, or illness. These are the hardest to think of because, while we try so hard to feel better, it feels ridiculous that part of us doesn't want to. This type of belief is usually in the format of *If I get better, then* _____ (insert with any negative aspect of healing you can think of; you may really have to stretch your mind to think of them).

Here are several examples of this: "If I get better, I'll be too overwhelmed with life;" "If I get better, I'll have to be intimate with my spouse again;" "If I get better, people will expect so much of me;" "If I get better, I'll have to go back to the job I hate;" "If I get better, I'll have no 'me time';" "If I get better, I'll lose financial support." If I were challenged to think of a hundred of these right now, I bet I could do it. That's how prevalent they are—so don't discount them just because they seem crazy.

Beliefs about Money

Beliefs about money drive us more than we are typically aware of, because money ties into our deep-rooted feelings about safety and security. I find that most people who "lack" well-being also have seriously limiting beliefs about money and not having enough. They are different topics or categories, but it's the same energy. In addition, because money can be related to our survival instinct, beliefs about money can have lots of tentacles—so they might also feel like they could fit into other categories. That's totally fine. The category doesn't matter at all, only that you identify them.

Examples: "Money is the root of all evil," "You can't have it all (money, love, and happiness)," "Rich people are bad or selfish people," "My parents struggled so I should too," "I'm unsafe when

I spend money," "I'm unlucky with money," "It's greedy to want money," "I'll never have enough money."

Beliefs about Relationships

This is all about our interactions with others, giving and receiving love and intimacy. Beliefs about relationships often tie into our self-esteem and what we believe others feel about us.

Examples: "No one will ever love me like _____ (a partner from the past, a parent, etc.)," "Getting close to someone is dangerous," "I will only get hurt," "I'm too messed up for someone to deal with," "Being in a relationship means I have to give up who I am," "Relationships always turn bad," "I can't trust anyone."

~~~

In making this list of your beliefs, did it become more clear that what you're believing is driving your life, and that those beliefs could be driving you *away* from feeling good? Because I was brought up with Yiddish-speaking family members, what most people experience as *aha* moments about beliefs were always huge *Oy veys!* for me.

Now you probably have a long list of target beliefs to work with. We can now start reprogramming you so that you can believe different things and have a new, healthier perspective on life. Remember that your brain runs much of your biology, so it's a fact that better things will come from your life when you believe better things. It's also just a more pleasant way to live day-to-day, right? Bonus.

How to Start to Change Your Beliefs

There are an endless number of beliefs to clear. Don't freak out about this. Even shifting a few of your harmful beliefs can make

a huge difference for you. Clearing these old beliefs can literally change the way you experience life without a single external
thing changing at all. I still constantly find and clear beliefs for
myself. It actually becomes kind of addicting after a while. It's a
game for me of *Let's see how crazy my brain actually is!* Seriously though,
they will be endless—and it doesn't matter. Just keep a running list in
your notebook and chip away at them slowly.

Start by picking out just a few beliefs from your list that feel most
relevant or connected to your depression. Once you check them
off the list, do a few more. Keep at it, and soon you will notice that
you've changed the way you experience life—for the better.

Note: When in part IV (chapter 10) you learn the advanced technique of muscle testing, you'll learn how to "test your work" to make
sure you successfully release the beliefs you're working on. But for
now, you can use your intuition. If you feel like you are still acting
from a place of believing a message, you may need to continue working on it and repeat the script a few more times. While muscle testing
can be quite helpful for this process, it's not absolutely necessary, so
let's start now.

An Extensive List of Beliefs

As promised, here's a long list of beliefs you may want to consider clearing. But don't feel like you need to do them all, or even
the majority of them, in order to feel better. You can also use the
muscle testing I teach you at the end of the book to narrow this list
down to beliefs that are most relevant to you. But you will be able
to tell by looking at a lot of them if you might need to clear them.
You can either copy them to your notebook or just put a check
mark right here on the pages.

With beliefs, it's most effective to tailor the phrase as close to your specific situation as possible. If my wording doesn't feel quite right to you, tweak it so it best describes what you believe.

The Ten Most Common Depression-Related Beliefs

If you can add a "because . . . " and elaborate just a bit, as in the first example that follows (for example, "because it's the only way I can say no"), it will be even more powerful for your healing.

I need this depression because _____ / If I heal _____ (insert downside here).

I deserve to / need to struggle.

I'm unsafe because _____.

I don't matter.

I need to stuff or suppress my emotions.

There's no point to feeling better.

I'm unlovable.

I don't deserve to be happy.

I am responsible for relieving the pain of others.

I'm not good enough.

Other Common Harmful Beliefs

The other shoe is always about to drop.

My life doesn't matter.

I have no purpose worth healing for.

I don't have permission to be happy.

This (energy therapy, medication, self-healing , etc.) won't work for me.

Expressing my emotions is dangerous.

If I feel my feelings, I'll die.

I can't handle life.

I deserve to be alone/unhappy/unhealthy.

I'll never get better or I'm unable to heal.

I'm destined to be depressed. (genetics)

I don't know how to feel good.

I need to be stuck to be safe.

I am delicate/weak.

The world is unsafe.

No one loves me.

Everything is my fault.

I'm too sensitive to be out in the world.

I'm broken.

I have to live my life for others.

I always make the wrong decision.

When things start to go well, something bad always happens.

If I do what I want, other people will be unhappy.

Being healthy and happy at the same time is impossible.

I'll only be loved if I'm perfect.

I have to hold all of my emotions in.

Depression is my punishment for doing something bad in the past.

Having depression is the only way I can say no to things I don't want to do.

I'll only be loved/taken care of if I am depressed.

It's unsafe to be my true self.

I deserve depression because I did something wrong in the past.

I'm undeserving of love.

I'm worthless.

Everyone else can heal, but I can't.

Overcoming depression is impossible.

Overcoming depression will take too much work.

I need this depression to have my needs met.

If I feel better, this will just happen again.

It's unsafe to be happy.

I'm not allowed to be happy.

I'm only worthy when _____ (I'm perfect, I'm doing things for others, etc.).

I need more money to feel better.

If I get well and still can't find a partner, I'll have no excuse.

Getting better would prove this was my fault in the first place.

I will be too vulnerable if I heal.

I'll have no idea what to do if I heal.

I have to forgive others or let them off the hook in order to feel better.

I will lose my identity if I feel better.

I'm too far behind in life to ever catch up.

I have to live up to others' (or my own) expectations.

I have to be perfect.

I'll have to be more assertive if I heal.

I'm not strong enough to get over this.

I need this depression as a distraction (from my unhappy life, my marriage, my job, etc.).

It will be unfair to the other people who are still suffering if I heal.

My life will change if I heal (and that's too scary).

I'll hurt my doctor's/friends'/family's feelings if I don't heal their way.

I'll have to be successful if I overcome this.

I'll lose my support system if I get better.

People will only believe I'm in pain if they see me suffering.

I've always had this problem and I always will.

I'm too damaged to heal.

Someone has to suffer, and maybe it's meant to be me.

My life will be too stressful if I'm healthy.

I'll have to be social if I heal.

I'll have to be present for my children if I heal.

Energy Therapy Exercise: Sweep Old Beliefs Away

You are going to say The Sweep script three times in a row while filling in the first blank with what you want to release (the negative belief). You can fill in the second blank (what you want to install) by using either the opposite belief of what you released or the simple general positive belief of "I can move forward with ease now."

Even though I have this _____ (belief that . . .), I acknowledge it's no longer working for me.

I give my subconscious full permission to help me clear it, from all of my cells in all of my body, permanently and completely.

I am now free to thank it for serving me in the past.

I am now free to release all resistances to letting it go.

I am now free to release all ideas that I need this in order to stay safe.

I am now free to release all ideas that I need it for any reason.

I am now free to release all feelings that I don't deserve to release it.

I am now free to release all conscious and subconscious causes for this energy.

I am now free to release all conscious and subconscious reasons for holding on to it.

I am now free to release all harmful patterns, emotions, and memories connected to it.

I am now free to release all generational or past-life energies keeping it stuck.

All of my being is healing and clearing this energy now, including any stress response stored in my cells.

Healing, healing, healing.

Clearing, clearing, clearing.

It is now time to install _____ (insert a new, healthy belief, for example, *I can move forward with ease now*).

Installing, installing, installing. Installing, installing, installing. And so it is done.

A note about installing positive beliefs: people get very hung up on what the "right" positive belief to install is. Simply try to think of the opposite message of what you just released and use that as your new belief. For example, if you released "I'll have to be social if I heal," a good opposite belief/message to install would be "I can heal no matter what" or "I can heal even if I want to keep to myself." One more example is if you released the belief "My life will change if I heal (and that's too scary)," a positive belief to install could be "I can handle changes in my life when I heal." Again, simply think of a healthier thing to believe and use that as your installation phrase. If you get stuck, use the general installation phrase I suggested in the script.

You should work on beliefs over time, as there will be too many to get to all at once. Just go slowly and remember that even a few can change your perspective on life entirely.

5

Deal with Your Feelings

Emotions are not logical. I argue this point to my clients on a regular basis. *Stop trying to figure them out,* I plead. *Stop adding so much freaking weight to them and let yourself just feel.* As humans, we spend so much time trying to figure out our emotions, control our emotions, judge our emotions *about* our emotions, and rationalize or talk ourselves out of our emotions just so we can appear stable, calm, and sane. In doing so, we inadvertently do the one thing we really should never do with our emotions: avoid or resist them. Yet, we all do it despite knowing—that in all the history of emotions—they have never gone away by simply ignoring them.

Here's the bottom line: you can't feel better by living your entire life stuck with emotions that make you feel like shit. But you also can't feel better by pretending they don't exist. The only way to deal with how you feel is to *deal* with how you feel. Or as the wise author and Buddhist teacher Sylvia Boorstein advises when it comes to our feelings, *Don't duck*. We must feel our emotions—and then process them out to heal them.

In this chapter, you're going to learn about the connection between emotions, thoughts, and feelings. You'll also discover why our emotions run our lives, and how you can work *with* them to feel better.

Emotions, First

We *feel* during 100 percent of our waking hours. And because emotions are essentially what we're made of, they influence every part of us, including our physical bodies. The word "emotion" comes from the Latin *emovēre*, "to disturb," which is from the Latin *e* + *movēre*, "to move." But when emotions or feelings that are considered "bad" are suppressed instead of allowed to move, we end up with prolonged feelings—making us *feel* really bad. In fact, suppressing emotions can easily trigger your body's *freakout* response because holding on to emotions is not natural and can feel dangerous or threatening to our system. We are not meant to feel everything indefinitely.

While it can seem like our emotions completely control us, that's not evidence that we should control them. Emotions are the absolute core of you—who you are, how you navigate the world, and what helps to create your individual experience in life. They are there to guide us, drive us, help us, and allow us to experience life. Art comes from emotion. Human connection comes from emotion. Fun comes from emotion. Emotions allow us to express ourselves and our needs. Suppressing your emotions will suppress your full and most joyous potential in all those areas of your life, and more. There is no way to be your true, unfettered self if you don't express how you feel.

The brain's limbic system is the emotional processing center; it sits behind the neocortex, the part of the brain in charge of conscious thoughts, reason, and decision-making. In a hierarchical sense of how we process life, emotions come first, almost instantly and involuntarily. They are not logical. From that emotion, we develop feelings (about the emotion). In this book, I use the terms "emotions" and "feelings" interchangeably, because while they technically have different biological meanings, they mean the same thing in terms of how we understand their role in our lives. So next, from how we feel, we create thoughts, which is essentially narration created by the mind about how we are feeling. This is how the mind attempts to explain what's going on—albeit usually not very well. Those thoughts then tend to create more feelings, and so the story goes.

Here's the tricky part. It's really hard to feel good when you're thinking shitty things. This is why the practice of changing your thoughts actually makes a whole lot of sense. This is also why it's complicated. Most of us achieve *not* having negative thoughts by ignoring the feelings driving them. But as we push them down, they push back against us, which can actually force us to focus on them. And whatever we focus on tends to have a light shone on it . . . meaning it gets amplified. So what are we to do? We know that not dealing with emotions (suppressing) hasn't worked, because that got us here in the first place. But we also know focusing on how bad you feel will not make you feel better, either (you've probably discovered this on your own). So, are we doomed? No. But it's now really clear why we can't just leave our mess as it is.

The best approach to helping you deal with all the things going on in yourself right now is to start with the emotions and feelings first; doing so can then change the trajectory of your thoughts in a more natural way. If you are currently practicing any of the popular "change your thoughts, change your life" programs and having success, please don't stop. But if you can't pull it off, I demand of you not to feel bad. Because, as you now understand, if we have to force you to think positively while you're feeling like shit, it will likely be an uphill battle. In that scenario, we are working in the wrong order of your brain's processing. When we start with the core of you—your emotions—you will naturally tend toward better-feeling thoughts. This way of going about things will be so much easier than trying to wrangle the constant narration driven by emotions we are trying to ignore.

We need to strike a balance of addressing emotions but not dwelling on them. When we get you even a tiny bit of relief from the heavy emotions you are burdened with, that's when you'll start feeling better. And when you start feeling better, it will be easier to find better-feeling thoughts more naturally, without forcing them.

You Are How You Feel: Why Emotions Matter

If you grew up in a house where intense emotions weren't allowed to be expressed or they were *too* freely expressed, the concept of dealing with your emotions might terrify you. You might have the belief that it's better not to deal with them at all. Maybe you feel that you are saving yourself from emotional pain. But as most of us learn eventually, suppressing how we feel doesn't save us anything at all. This MO morphs into an automatic response that operates unknowingly behind the scenes of your life, squashing your ability to feel good.

Many healing approaches teach us to "master," "control," or simply become "aware" of our emotions. Some offer the suggestions to "think positive" or "change your thoughts" in order to feel better things. And no one can argue that being aware of our emotions or thinking more positively isn't a good thing. But there are a few reasons why these methods aren't the cure-all for feeling like shit.

First, awareness is not always the key. Although talk therapy can be beneficial by helping us understand how we feel, because emotions are often illogical, we may end up in therapy for years without solving the mystery of why we feel the way we do or finding resolution. In addition, just because we understand our feelings doesn't mean we always let them go from our body. When emotions are lodged in the body but not dealt with, we can end up feeling them all of the time with no relief (even if we are lucky enough to understand *why* we feel them).

Second, it's an impossibly exhausting task to keep the positivity train going all the darn time. No one can feel or be positive all the time, or even most of the time—especially when you feel bad. Because in a twist of cruelty, the worse we *feel*, the worse we feel. There's that momentum we've been talking about. Because you now understand that emotion and feeling come first in a chronological sense of how things work, I'm going to help you make sense of something big: you simply cannot *think* your way out of bad feelings. You must deal with the feeling in order to feel and think better. Everything in healing and feeling good falls back on having effective ways to deal with your feelings.

Finally, here's what's most important to know. When we lack the tools to deal with our emotions and they become too painful to bear, it's no wonder we suppress them in an effort to avoid them. But when we're "turned off" to our pain, we are actually turned off to all feelings—the "bad" and the "good." There is no way to cherry-pick only the emotions that you want to feel. If you don't allow the undesirable, you're automatically disallowing what you do want too: joy, contentment, and happiness. If you push away even some "bad" emotions, you will inadvertently push away some "good" ones too.

When everything is stuffed down, we can even lose the capacity to feel our emotions fully, creating a lack of awareness about when we are experiencing stress or about what we need in life to survive and thrive. In addition, trying to control anything will play into your body's fight, flight, or freeze response. This actually causes stress, which triggers you into *freakout* mode. And at this point, you totally understand that being in *freakout* mode can contribute to subconscious sabotage . . . and depression.

Emotions are part of our precious built-in survival and navigation systems. If you manipulate your emotions, you are quite literally manipulating who you are and your experience and direction in life. We often try to control our emotions in the name of being better or happier people. But what if we are manipulating ourselves away from our truest, best selves?

Can you now see why trying to feel better while also trying to control your emotions is almost impossible? If you're thinking, *What a mess!*, you're on point. But don't worry, there's a method to wrangle all this emotional madness, and I'm going to help you learn it.

Trying to control emotions is the single most detrimental thing you can do, but it's often our first go-to. Let's delve deeper into an important aspect of what drives this behavior.

The Role of Vulnerability

Emotions are the primary way we connect with others. In fact, for all the ways we perceive that sharing our emotions causes trouble, it's actually worse for us not to. Sharing our truest, most vulnerable selves actually prevents us from the isolation that occurs when we miss out on the deep connection that only comes from this type of transparency. While social media can be a place of great support, it's also caused a huge challenge. Because we've created a world in which we are addicted to showing our curated emotions, social media posts rarely tell the entire story. We've gotten accustomed to holding back our real selves—so much, in fact, that we have a totally distorted view of what's "real."

On a wet fall day as I was researching the negative effects of social media for this book, I noticed that a heavy sense of melancholy had fallen over me. Pushing myself to go out for a short walk in my beloved Central Park, only a block away, took every ounce of energy I had. When I was out, my sadness didn't fade, but astounded by the colorful change of leaves, I felt inspired to take a handful of photos. They were the kind that Instagram is made of. When I got home, I decided to post them on social media. But earlier that day I had read something that was still with me: what happened when Tracy Clayton, host of the BuzzFeed podcast *Another Round*, asked people to repost photos they'd previously shared on social media, but this time, with the "real story" behind them. The photos that most of us would have longed for had painful stories behind them. One woman admitted to a terrible anxiety attack that took her all day to overcome, someone else shared the grief over a loss of a loved one stuffed under their smile at a party, and so on. What this shows us is that we are all running after a farce. But what's worse, it shows that we're all co-creating it.

So after a brief pause, I posted my gorgeous fall photos from the park with this: *Full disclosure: Inspired by research for my next book about how social media posts screw us up by making everything and everyone seem OK even when they are not, I'm adding the truth here. These pictures were taken on a walk I dragged myself on because I felt sad today for no particular reason (except for that life is a lot sometimes).*

I am typically not a sad person, nor am I one who shares it on social media when I am. I am very transparent on my author account, but for some reason, I am less so on my personal page. The response that day when I shared how I really felt took me by great surprise. Dozens of people I rarely heard from came out of the blue with comments, texts, and private messages. And what most of them were saying was, "I feel that way too." In our technological age, we are more connected than ever before, but also lonelier and more isolated than ever before. I wondered that day, *What if everyone stopped staying so busy pretending everything was perfect? What if instead of hiding our vulnerabilities to prevent the isolation we fear, we are driving it?*

The bottom line is that, over and over again, I've learned that emotions are better in every way when they aren't kept inside and to myself. But let's talk about how to deal with not even trusting your own feelings enough to accept them.

When It's Hard to Trust How You Feel

Do you ever find yourself thinking, *I don't even know how I feel anymore!* If you have long been in the practice of stuffing emotions and/or paying more attention to how you think you should feel based on society's or others' opinions (cut to social media), you may feel very little or feel several conflicting things. Losing track of how we feel typically happens when (1) we talk ourselves out of feeling how we really do, or (2) we're too afraid to face it. It can be inconvenient to feel how we feel sometimes. In fact, maybe you've had the experience of other people in your life talking you out of how you felt (or calling you crazy or unhinged) because it was inconvenient for *them*.

Either of these scenarios can lead to emotions that seem all over the place or exaggerated. If this sounds like you, and you often find yourself wondering what's even real, know that this is so common.

I want you to know that you can trust how you feel—even if you don't like it, don't understand it, or it seems irrational. Feelings are never fake, but emotions can become intensified and complex when they are *not moving*. This can make them feel confusing, crazy, unreal, and unpredictable. Even if you feel like you are overreacting to something emotionally, it's essential that you honor it because it's real for you (and likely a clue to what you're feeling on a deep level). A feeling is no less relevant just because you can't figure it out. If it's there, for whatever reason, it's relevant. When I work with kids, they sometimes tell me how they feel and why they feel that way, and I immediately recognize what they are upset about might not have really happened ("My teddy bear pushed me out of the way and stole my toy!") or they are reacting on a skewed perception ("My mom hates me because she won't get me new shoes!"). But I help them deal with their feelings as they are. I accept their feelings as 100 percent true and real because that's the only way we can get them to move through. And you have to do the same. You must honor your feelings because they are the *reality* of how you feel.

I always used to make excuses to not trust or believe my own emotions because they didn't make sense, but the illogical eruptions of emotions are usually the biggest truths begging to be heard. Because I used to work so hard to suppress everything I felt, most of my emotions that actually made it to the surface were intense, dramatic, and felt uncontrollable. Looking back, this actually did make total sense. I see this pattern most with people like me who tend toward perfectionism and type A personality traits, those who worry about how they appear to others and who hold themselves to impossible expectations. This is just how the expression manifests because of the coping mechanism of suppression.

I sometimes joke that if you want to know what emotions you're really harboring inside, observe yourself when you've had an alcoholic drink or have PMS. It'll all be extremely obvious. We often blame these scenarios for why we got "out of control," but it's actually that those situations tend to magnify what's already there that needs to be acknowledged. I'm certainly not suggesting you use hormones and alcohol to test how you really feel deep down, but it's interesting to understand how certain things can highlight what we feel and what we aren't dealing with.

A Note About Feelings from the Past

We often perceive that our feelings are "current"—about what our boss just did, how frustrated we feel with our spouse, and more—but the majority of the emotions we feel are old, from the past but still active within us. Remember that unexpressed emotions are literally lodged in the body. When we haven't dealt with emotional baggage from the past in the form of trauma (as we'll be doing in the next chapter), the feelings we have may get triggered from *then* but show up *now*. In other words, how we feel now is a resonance of what we've felt before, just being activated in the present moment. When we don't deal with traumas from the past, the individual emotions from them continue to come up again and again until we do something about them. Though our current emotions may be rooted in the past, they are still very real. They still have context in your body that validates why you feel how you do; they are simply distanced from the actual point of origin. This makes things very confusing and often leaves us perplexed as to why we feel how we do, even when things seem to be going just fine. This is maybe what's going on consciously, but what's happening behind the scenes may tell a different story.

In this chapter, we're going to focus on how we feel now—regardless of why or how it came to be. In the next chapter, we'll go back to clean up the old stuff that's still hanging out in your body. But because our current experience is inexplicably connected to the past, we're unconsciously working on both.

For now, we need to first learn how to deal with the here and now so we stop perpetuating this unhealthy cycle of suppression and depression. In addition, dealing with our emotions in our current state can help us start to feel better as we work on the stuff from the past. Because while dealing with the past is totally doable, it can be a lengthy process—although, thankfully, it's not agonizing like you might be imagining.

Find Emotional Relief

Although we soon will go back to deal with your past, which will help enormously in how you feel *now*, we need a place to start, a way to cleanse ourselves of the feelings occupying our current space. Your past is only affecting you now because you have accumulated more emotional energy than your body can hold.

Our bodies are like pots of boiling water. If we continuously keep the lid on ourselves, never letting out any of the steam, the pressure is going to overwhelm us. But if we find a way to let out a small amount of pressure as it arises, we are able to hold our center without exploding.

To begin, we have to stop stuffing down, tucking away, or postponing how we feel until we "have time" or energy to deal with it. The idea behind dealing with emotions is not to learn to cope with them but to release or *move* the energy that's been stuck so that *you* can move on. Through the process of dealing with your emotions, you are actually teaching your body a new pattern: *letting go* of your feelings instead of *holding on* to them. When I began working in this way, I enjoyed the unexpected side effect of naturally letting go of emotions faster without trying. Prior to that, I described myself as the girl who could hold a grudge over one misspoken word—for years. Now, I joke, I only hold it for approximately three months . . . or if I'm really lucky, three days.

You may have tried previous approaches that promised to get you to go from feeling bad to feeling good or happy right away—and failed. We're going to have a different goal here: emotional relief. Because of the concept of momentum, you now understand that if we can get you to feel a little better, you can feel a little better from there, and on and on.

All you need to do is practice this simple process: allow your feelings to come up (without a bunch of extra stuff like judgment, shame, or resistance) *while* using the energy exercise we'll be doing shortly to let them go from your body. The key to getting emotional relief is to not add a whole bunch of emotions about your emotions in the process of having emotions! You'll be using this process (allow + release) whenever you can throughout the day, especially when you are feeling strong emotion or feeling really bad. Even if the emotions you feel are linked to another person or an unchangeable situation, it doesn't matter. The very best thing you will ever do for yourself is to deal with the way you feel without trying to change (the possibly unchangeable thing) that you have so many feelings *about*. This is your ticket to freedom: to give up the never-ending chore of trying to control everything.

Your only responsibility is to get the feelings out of your body so that you can find emotional relief. By simply addressing the way you feel, without trying to change anything else right

now, better days are on your horizon. The good news is that
it's not terribly hard and actually becomes an automatic habit
once you start. In fact, you are already going to great lengths
not to feel bad in many ways—using addictions, suppression, or
whatever it may be. This new process will be easier than that.
But it can only work if you do it. There's no way around it: you
cannot feel better while trying to suppress emotions that make
you feel like shit.

Now, let's talk about which specific emotions might be helpful
to focus on as a start.

The "Big Three" Emotions

You won't know what you need to let go of unless you learn to
identify how you really feel. One of the things people have become
really good at is dumping their feelings into general categories of
"depression" or "anxiety." How often do you repeat *I'm depressed*
without even giving thought to what that means or what might be
under it? The true gold in working with emotions is to first identify
how you really feel. "Depression" is a way to describe it, yes, but
depression doesn't exist on its own.

Often, especially when it comes to energy work, people will say
to me that they aren't sure what to work on or what they are feeling. This is normal, because we typically go to that fallback of *I feel
depressed*. But there's a method to the madness of discovering what
energies you might need to work on.

While humans suppress and ignore a range of emotions that
can then become stuck, there are three that I've found to hold the
most weight, often because how we feel about them and tend to
process them is not straightforward. I call these emotions "the big
three": anger, grief, and fear. You might be thinking that you are

already familiar with these emotions, but let's talk a little bit about them to give you a new window into what they truly mean. We are going to use these three as our starting point in dealing with our feelings.

Anger

Anger is easily the most ignored and disguised emotion there is, especially for women. For a lot of people, anger seems the scariest, most out of control, ugly, and against the rules. If you grew up in a violent household, it can be most closely connected to your trauma from childhood. In addition, very sensitive people are often terrified of anger either within themselves or with others. Because some of us have the idea that we'd be bad or mean people if we felt angry, we are desperate not to *become* angry. But in that, this very natural and necessary emotion gets stifled. I always insisted I wasn't an angry person, even after I learned how much anger plays a role in our physical health. But what I realized is that anger is very disguised. For instance, do you tend to cry in frustration when you're angry at someone or about something? Or do you retreat into sadness and want to be alone? Or even get silently resentful and find yourself with scary feelings of hatred and resentment for others? If so, you have likely been suppressing anger. Realizing how I dealt with anger helped snap me into reality about it—I was angry and resentful inside; it just didn't manifest like we imagine anger does. I often acted out my anger with those who had hurt me by punishing them—withholding intimacy, cutting them off emotionally, or finding other ways to show them they were wrong. I also ignored a major source of anger for myself: self-hatred, wrapped up in my ridiculous expectations of myself. Anger often comes out sideways—as sadness (because we can't express how we truly feel), as pain or inflammation in the body, and as passive-aggressive behaviors. When we are so desperate to avoid anger, we can unintentionally give it more "life" than it would have otherwise.

A note about forgiveness: there is an entire industry built around the idea of healing through forgiveness. But I don't buy into any of it, except in one case: self-forgiveness. I don't believe—and have not seen—that you must forgive anyone else in order to move on. But you must find a way to dispel the anger within yourself in order to be at peace. I find this important to say because while everyone is running around trying to force themselves to forgive people in their life, they are sometimes mistakenly further suppressing anger. So I'm stating it here loud and clear: you do not need to forgive to heal. But you do need to release the anger from your body, especially if it's self-directed.

Grief

Grief is the emotion perhaps most directly connected to depression. We often think of grief as related to a death or major loss, but where we go wrong is limiting our definition of it. We demand that grief is only warranted when we lose a loved one, suffer a misfortune that ruins our lives, or experience a disaster that's irreparable. But grief—grieving—is a natural part of life. And if we push it down, it breeds hopelessness. It is one of the trickiest emotions to deal with, though, because it is unpredictable, confusing, and can linger. Grief is something that we don't often "have time for," especially once we've passed the "acceptable time of grieving" or had to go back to daily life after a period of respite. Think of how many times you've choked back tears in public, because bursting into tears over a loss isn't exactly socially acceptable. It's been almost ten years since my dad died, and I still have waves of grief that bowl me over at the most inconvenient times.

Humans grieve over everything, death being the most accepted. But we also grieve for our disappointments and expectations (for example, a friend who doesn't support you), or loss of time or life (in the case of a chronic illness, all the things you didn't get to do or be), or changed life or relationships (a move or divorce), and things we wanted for our lives that didn't happen (having children, getting to travel, and more). Grief is easily glossed over because we are hesitant to be vulnerable by grieving over something that doesn't seem like "a big deal." I always say that we have the most grief over the things we have no time to grieve. And depression is a common way we grieve, silently, for needs unmet or a life unfulfilled.

Fear

Fear may seem like an emotion that's relatively acceptable to have and even share. Fear is the emotion often linked to impending danger, pain (emotional or physical), or intimidation. It is easy to understand and have compassion for. But fear runs so much deeper than the simple response to threats. Fear is one of the most complex human emotions because it often rocks the very essence of who we are. Fear can be divided into two main categories: fear of being unsafe (emotionally or physically), and fear of being unloved. Every fear—from the common fear of heights to the fear of sharing feelings—will be connected to one or both of these. But there is one greatest fear that creates the most havoc in our lives, and it's the most commonly ignored: the fear of being who we really are. The fear of being our true selves is a relentless fear that, if not dealt with, is a driving force in the suppression and behaviors that lead to depression. Being who we are without apology or manipulation is what allows us to meet the needs of our lives— physically, emotionally, and spiritually. Without this, we simply

cannot inhabit our full joy. It's impossible to do so while you are
blocking the essence of it: the true you.

~~~

Are you thinking about "the big three" in a new way now? Can
you think of what you might be angry, grieving, or fearful about
(especially related to who you really are) that you haven't allowed
yourself to express?

Let's talk a little bit about what we'll be doing together now
that (hopefully) helps you see the importance of working with your
anger, grief, fear, and other feelings.

When to Deal with Your Feelings

We are going to start dealing with feelings by deciding, once and
for all, to just do it. Because, as you remember, *it only takes feeling
a little better to have better feelings*. Dealing with emotions is super
straightforward: we need to feel our feelings fully while using
the techniques I'm going to teach you. Then, rinse and repeat
for the rest of your life. It may sound like a lot of work, but it's
not. I promise you've been using more energy trying to avoid
your feelings than you will be by dealing with them. Pretty soon,
this process will be automatic. *Feel bad → use technique for relief. Feel
bad → use technique for relief. Feel bad → use technique for relief.* There is
no reason you'll have to suppress anymore, because you'll know
exactly what to do with uncomfortable feelings to help move them
through you more naturally and fully.

This process should be used whenever you feel like shit—from
feeling sad for "no reason" to being angry because something feels
unfair, and everything in between. Think of these tools as a way
to help move your feelings along a little faster. If you are sitting

around feeling bad, you might as well be sitting around using the techniques to get relief. You don't need to sit for hours, although dealing with our feelings may take some time. But even five- to ten-minute intervals can make a huge difference.

Identify Which Emotions to Address

Now, how to know what to deal with first? This is easier than you may think. I'm going to guide you. You can use the process of *feel bad → use technique for relief* for any single emotion, or for lots of feelings and random thoughts you're having at once, even if they make zero logical sense. When deciding what to deal with, you can also think about these questions: *What would you complain about to a friend if they called right now? What thoughts are taking up space in your brain? Which of "the big three" do you resonate with right now?* By asking yourself these questions in the moment, you'll be able to best identify what you need to work with at any given time.

Each time you sit down to deal with your feelings, you may answer the question differently. That's totally good! Whatever you want to work on letting go of is a great choice.

Remember, we'll be dealing with trauma from our past in the next chapter, which will give you more to work with.

Energy Therapy Exercises: Two Ways to Deal with Your Feelings

When you are at the point of simply dealing with your present emotions, the explanation behind the emotions doesn't matter. Whenever you feel bad, you are feeling something that's being triggered. And the best way to relieve that feeling is to acknowledge, process, and release it. I'm going to give you two techniques to do this: Tapping, and Thymus Test and Tap (TTT). They each work differently, so I like to use them both—sometimes one or the other depending on how I'm feeling. But using them together will give you a synergistic effect that helps you feel better even faster.

Tapping to Deal with Stuck Emotions

Use this tapping script to help you work through how you feel . . . and let those emotions go. Again, you can focus on one specific emotion you're feeling (for example, anger or one of the other "big three" that you identify with strongly) or a general myriad of feelings (basically, all the random thoughts and feelings you have). And even if you start with one thing and then start feeling another, that's okay. You can switch and go back and forth at any time. Remember that tapping is largely a process of "venting," so don't put any pressure on yourself about what is the "right" way to describe how you feel. Some examples of phrases that could describe how you feel are:

* Feeling like shit

* Angry that I'm still depressed even though I try so hard

* Upset that my dad is mad at me

* Scared about my future

We are simply looking for how you describe how you feel. It can be anything!

I'm going to give you some great prompts in the following tapping script, but you can stray from the script and go rogue too. That will only make it even more effective because it'll be personalized to you.

You are free to use any set of tapping points you'd like (you learned three ways to tap in chapter 3), but you will start with the karate-chop point no matter what.

As a reminder, here are the tapping points for each of the three techniques. Remember, you only need to choose one to work with.

Temple Tapping Points: At your temples on each side. If you only have the physical use of one hand, you can use that hand to tap the temples alternately.

Emotional Freedom Technique Points: Top of the head—*Tapping point:* This is smack dab in the middle of the top of your head. Eyebrow—*Tapping point:* The inside corner of the eye, right where the eyebrow starts. Side of the eye—*Tapping point:* The outer corner of the eye, right on the bone, close to where it meets your temple. Under the eye—*Tapping point:* The top of the cheekbone, right under the eye. Top lip—*Tapping point:* This is where a mustache would be if you had one. Chin—*Tapping point:* In the indentation on your chin, halfway between your bottom lip and the tip of your chin. Collarbone—*Tapping point:* Find where you would tie a tie on your neck, then go out to the side an inch and drop directly under the collarbone. Under the arm/side of the body—*Tapping point:* This is where a bra band is, about four inches under the armpit on the side of the body. Fingertips—*Tapping points:* The lower right-hand corner of each fingernail, where it meets the cuticle. You only need to tap on the fingertips of one hand.

Chakra Tapping Points: Crown (Seventh) Chakra—*Tapping Point:* Top of the head. Third Eye or Brow (Sixth) Chakra—*Tapping Point:* In between the eyebrows. Throat (Fifth) Chakra—*Tapping Point:* Front of the throat. Heart (Fourth) Chakra—*Tapping Point:* In the middle of the chest. Solar Plexus (Third) Chakra—*Tapping Point:* Right under the sternum at your solar plexus. Sacral (Second) Chakra—*Tapping Point:* Just below the belly button. Root (First) Chakra—*Tapping Point:* Top of your thighs (pat them like you're calling a puppy up on your lap).

Step 1: Start tapping on the karate-chop point continuously while repeating these statements:

Even though I feel _____ (describe or summarize the problem in a couple of sentences), *I choose to let it go.*

Even though I feel _____, *I choose to let it go.*

Even though I feel _____, *I can be okay anyway.*

Step 2: Cycle through the rest of the points using these statements as a guide (add your own or revise mine to feel more natural):

I feel _____.

I keep thinking about or worrying about _____.

I feel it in my _____ (name part of body if you feel the emotion somewhere).

I feel _____.

I don't know what to do.

I just keep feeling _____.

I feel _____ *about it* (sometimes identifying how you feel about a problem, like "mad" or "frustrated," helps to diffuse it).

It feels like _____ (describe it in detail—scary, annoying, achy, etc.).

I am really struggling with _____.

You are simply "venting" about how you feel here, so any phrases that feel true for you will work. Remember, it can be anything you think or feel about it. No one else will ever know what you say or think.

Continue tapping for several more rounds, tapping through all the points while "venting" about how you feel. Incorporate any ideas or thoughts that pop up for you. Take a deep breath or two between every few rounds.

Step 3: Wrap up with positive statements. Once you are happy with the improvement or are done with your tapping session, do one more round using all positive statements. You can choose any of the following:

I'm releasing old energy now.

I can be okay now.

I am safe.

That's it! The more you use this, the more comfortable you'll get. Just remember, all you have to do is bring up your feelings (by talking or thinking about them), and tap at the same time.

Now, let's learn another totally different way to deal with your emotions.

Thymus Test and Tap (TTT) to Release Individual Stuck Emotions

As I mentioned earlier in the chapter, a lot of what we feel *now* is because we still have feelings that are unprocessed from the past. The problem is that those feelings aren't always obvious to us. You'll learn a lot more about this soon, but for now, using TTT can release even emotions that you aren't consciously aware of. I love sitting down to use this when I'm feeling bad because it helps me access things I am not consciously tuned in to. And a lot of times, that's exactly what we need.

| THYMUS TEST AND TAP (TTT) UNPROCESSED EMOTIONS ||
Section 1	Section 2
Abandoned	Helpless
Fearful	Hopeless
Grief-stricken	Heavy
Unloved	Impatient
Intimidated	Out of control
Criticized	Defensive
Judged	Frustrated
Hated	Panicked
Berated	Insecure
Worthless	Powerless
Attacked	Shocked
Betrayed	Failure
Disconnected	Stressed
Section 3	Section 4
Rejected	Vulnerable
Angry	Unsupported
Guilty	Undeserving
Resentful	Ashamed
Blamed	Overwhelmed
Indecisiveness	Bullied
Disgusted	Lonely
Conflicted	Alone
Confused	Regretful
Nervous	Disappointed
Unsafe	Discarded
Worried	Excluded
Hurt	Desperate
Resistant	Traumatized

This technique allows us to zoom in on and identify emotions stuck in our body and then release them one by one as we tap the thymus gland. I often release ten or twenty emotions in one sitting, but even releasing just a few can make a huge difference. You may want to "start small" since this is your first time. You'll have to gauge intuitively when to stop.

Step 1: Identify an emotion to work with. Sit quietly and ask yourself which emotion on the list might be coming up in your current situation. You can also ask what emotion is making you feel "depressed" (or "exhausted," "confused," "overwhelmed," or anything else you want to address). Now, close your eyes and gently swirl your pointer finger all over the list of emotions. You can make big circles or any shape you want, but try to cover the entire list. When you feel called to stop, stop while holding your finger in place. This is your body intuitively picking up on the emotion you need to release. (Remember, you can muscle test for the emotions, too, which we'll discuss in chapter 10).

Step 2: Tap your thymus gland seven times repetitively to release. Now that you have identified the first emotion stuck in your body, you are ready to tap your thymus to let it go. Simply tap at least seven times firmly over your thymus gland with the finger-tips of one hand. (You may want to look back to chapter 3 to see where your thymus gland is.) We are using this tapping percussion to flush the stuck energy out of your system. I like to say, *Releasing, releasing, releasing* or *Let go, let go, let go* as I tap. Tap as many times as you need in order to feel like you've released the emotion. If you don't feel anything, know that seven is plenty.

Step 3: Take a deep breath and begin all over. This is a process you can sit down to do anytime you're dealing with tough feelings. Not only will it help you feel more comfortable with how you feel, but it will be reversing that long-held pattern of stifling emotions that contributes to depression. Hooray. You're going to start feeling so much better by doing this regularly.

Now, let's take a little trip back to your past to see what we can address there to truly clear out some major roots of why you've been feeling so bad.

6

Heal Trauma from the Past

While we'd all like to think we aren't products of our past, it's hard not to function as if we are. And it's no wonder. When something distressing happens in our lives, it makes sense that it becomes part of us and affects our lives. You have probably heard—and maybe tried—a million times, to *deal with trauma* and *let go of your past*. Maybe you've been to therapy and hashed out every detail of whatever you remember from your life that went wrong. You might even have a better understanding or perspective of how your past has influenced you. But what if telling and retelling your story hasn't helped you actually move on? Or worse, what if doing so has only made it more part of your life? Trauma can be a confusing topic, so maybe you don't even know what you're supposed to be letting go of anymore, or how to do it.

It is indeed important to address our past and its traumas, but it has to be done in a way that settles it instead of stirs it. Sometimes, healing trauma is, in part, to come to peace with the *not making sense* of it. It may be only then that your heart and body can stop rehashing it and rest.

This chapter is going to help you not only *see* trauma in a new way but also *address* it in a new way. I will also help you understand what you can do in the future to prevent trauma—and if it happens, how to keep it from having such a hold on your life.

The Root of Trauma: Unprocessed Experiences

Trauma is something that you've probably heard a lot about, especially in the past few years, because science has caught up to explaining how trauma is involved in conditions from depression to chronic illness and pain. It can feel like such a big, scary word, but it's often misunderstood. Many people think of trauma as massive life-altering events such as abuse, neglect, death, or an accident. In fact, for this reason, I've tended to shy away from using the word "trauma" in my work, as it can be jarring in itself. But over the years, I've realized that unless we call it trauma, people don't recognize it as something "big enough" to honor and address. So I'm going to call it by its name but also help you understand why it's not always so big and scary.

It's interesting to note here that emotions, trauma, and beliefs are all connected—as if they are tangled up in the same web. As you work with each piece, you're likely resolving a lot more than you realize. When people go through distressing situations and don't discharge their feelings, those emotions can end up getting stuck inside of us. These experiences that remain unprocessed become part of what form those pesky beliefs (or takeaway messages) that cause so much trouble in our lives. So by releasing unprocessed experiences and the connected emotions, you are also continuing to work on beliefs that might be blocking you from feeling good.

How Trauma Happens

Because of how much our modern lifestyles require of us (and how we require so much of ourselves), our system often can't distinguish between stress from an actual threat and stress from past unresolved emotional experiences. It just detects "stress" and reacts accordingly. Trauma happens when we go through certain *experiences* in our lives and are not able to *process* and let go of them. Trauma can be linked to "big" events as well as to events that seem meaningless or "small"—yet still had a negative impact on you. The common denominator in trauma is that you have not processed and let go of your emotions surrounding the event. I call these events *unprocessed experiences*. These are snapshots of time, or memories, such as "when Dad died" or "that time Mom forgot me at school." Experiences are essentially memories that get stored in the body as feelings, "movies," or images. I see trauma as the emotional energy from any experience that is unresolved within yourself—in other words, unfinished with your mind, body, or spirit. It's super important to know that not every seemingly traumatic experience will traumatize you (which we'll talk more about soon). In fact, here's the thing: the majority of experiences that I see contribute to depression are experiences that people have not yet addressed or talked about, because they seemed "too small" or "silly" to negatively affect them. While we tend to share big traumas and get help to find peace around them, the smaller or unimportant things get neglected and stuck in our bodies, affecting our entire lives. In fact, experiences that seem more "minor" in the big picture of life—from witnessing a fight between your parents to being teased in kindergarten—can actually be more traumatizing than the biggies because of our dismissal of them. In addition, trauma often occurs not because of the gravity of the situation or event itself, but because it happens at an age or time when we don't possess the mental and emotional capacity, or have appropriate skills, to deal with it.

It's essential to understand that everyone has trauma in their body—and quite possibly, a lot of it. Just like having lots of emotions, it's actually quite normal. Not all "negative" events create trauma, because as you know, each person responds to experiences differently. And not all trauma is going to cause depression. There's no need to judge or berate yourself for what you've been holding on to. The whole point of this work is to let go—not create more trauma by beating yourself up.

Now that we've gotten that out of the way, let's talk about why it's so important to not just try to "forget the past." You might already have some ideas of what parts of your past you need to deal with just from going through those general parameters of trauma. We're going to be talking about trauma in more detail soon. For now, keep a running list of ideas or events from your past as you think of them; later in the chapter I'll help you work with them.

It's important to know that trauma is not just about what happened to you, it's also about what happened *within* you— specifically your energy system at the time of the experience. Let's take a closer look.

The Bzzzt: *Trauma and the Energy System*

Energetically speaking, trauma all comes down to one little *bzzzt* that occurs in the energy system during some stressful life events.

This phenomenon is part of how Gary Craig, creator of the Emotional Freedom Technique (EFT), discovered the effectiveness of tapping when releasing trauma. Let me explain how this plays out.

Imagine that you and your brother have the same experience of being embarrassed at school—for example, being called out by the teacher in front of class for getting an "easy" math problem wrong. It could be that you get really affected by it and end up in tears while your brother shrugs it off. Maybe you continue to recall it and relive it throughout your life, getting sweaty palms every time you have to speak in a group, yet your brother never thinks about it again. This difference in how each of you is affected can be explained by what is happening in the energy system at the time of emotional stress. Let's imagine that while you are having this stressful experience, your energy system reacts by experiencing a little *electrical zap (hzzzt)*, which disrupts your energy flow throughout your system and causes an imbalance or "block." Your brother's energy system does not react in this way, so his energy continues to flow as it should.

If we get that little short circuit, or *bzzzt*, in our energy system, the emotional experience is more likely to get stuck and have a lasting effect on us. Whether or not this happens to an individual is not predictable, but rather a matter of each person's individual energy system. I believe that those of us with sensitive nervous systems have a greater tendency for our energy flow to get disrupted or imbalanced during such experiences. This means we may be more likely to get traumatized. However, those of us who tend to have more traumas lean toward more delicate nervous systems, perpetuating this pattern. So it's a little bit of a "chicken or egg" scenario. It's also become clear to me that those of us who tend to hold on to things consciously (such as who did what to them, unpleasant memories, and more) also tend to hold on ener-getically—and vice versa. You'll remember how I told you that I can be a grudge holder? I believe that part of my personality lends itself to the pattern of hanging on to things in my physical body too long. As I've worked to reverse this pattern mentally, things have shifted energetically. I have definitely noticed a link between those people who tend to fixate or analyze and those who tend to hold on energetically. None of this is bad, but it does give us a new way to understand why trauma happens and how to deal with it.

This explanation of how different people are affected by the same experience helps us understand even more how experiences can be *traumatizing*, even if we wouldn't immediately consider them *traumatic*. This is why so many people come to me professing that nothing "*that* bad" has ever happened to them, so they don't understand why they feel like shit. It's easy to let an experience like the school incident slip under the radar. But how many of us have experienced something similar? Probably everyone has, in one way or another. So if we ignore stressful experiences like this and brush off their potential impact, the depression we feel can seem dispro-portionate to our lives. Another thing I hear often is that someone has spent years in therapy and the trauma is not going away. But if we look at trauma as connected to our energy system, we can easily see why talk therapy or behavioral therapy alone may not heal trauma. We may need to address the energy system and get rid of that *bzzzt* to truly resolve and heal it.

Some experiences that contribute to depression will be ones we remember, and some we won't. I'll be helping you address both. But for now, a good way to explore how unprocessed experiences might feel in your body is to briefly recall a memory from your past and see if you have an emotional "charge" associated with that memory. An emotional charge is typically an uncomfortable sensation in your body, such as a pit in your stomach, tightness in your shoulder, or a flushed feeling. That charge you are feeling is essentially the *bzzzt* that occurs within the energy system. Simply put, it's the disruption of your energy flow in relationship to (or when you think about) that memory.

Energy therapy gives us a way to heal that zap in the energy system that contributed to trauma in the first place. The really cool thing is that the more we balance our energy system through releasing trauma and healing our emotions, the less likely we are to be effected in such a negative way by distressing experiences in the future—because we'll be setting that pattern of letting go while strengthening our system.

The Trauma-Trigger Cycle

When you are stuck with old unprocessed experiences living inside you, they can create what I call a trauma-trigger cycle because they are still very much alive in our systems.

Here's my analogy to help you understand how this works and why it causes so much trouble. Imagine that you have a very difficult experience, for example, having to say goodbye to a sick pet. All of the details in the form of individual feelings, smells, images, sounds, and more get bundled up and deposited into a metaphorical glass *trauma capsule*—which gets stored in the body. It sits there with all of the old feelings we experienced at the time the event happened. While you might not be aware of it constantly, you are likely feeling those emotions at a low level all the time. When any current situation reminds you of any of those details hanging out in the capsule—either consciously or subconsciously—the old trauma gets "poked," or reactivated. This is how we get *triggered*.

Being triggered can bring up flashes of those memories, including images, feelings, and any sensory stimuli.

For the most part, except in certain cases of post-traumatic stress disorder (PTSD) from major life events, where sometimes the trigger is known, this trauma-trigger reaction actually happens at a subconscious level, outside of your awareness. Even in obvious situations, you may think you know what the trigger is, and try to avoid it, but it may be something totally different that got stuck in the metaphorical glass trauma capsule. Often, people come to me and say, "Nothing set this off," "I'm depressed for no reason," or "I suddenly started feeling terrible but nothing happened." While this may seem true, I can bet on the fact that while the bad feelings might seem random, they are being triggered in some way that you simply haven't yet identified. Triggers can be foods, colors, smells, sounds, weather, or anything, really! Finding and resolving triggers can become almost an entertaining game if you let it. I'll be teaching you how to address specific triggers in chapter 11, once you've mastered the basics of working with unprocessed experiences.

As you can imagine, this entire trauma-trigger dynamic is very unsettling and unpredictable—which can feel like danger to your system and keep you stuck in that *freakout* response. Not only that, but in this state, you can actually be excessively tuned in to your trauma, seeing reminders of it everywhere, which further traumatizes you.

I had an experience after going through a loved one's difficult health crisis where every single place I looked, I saw reminders of the experience. And for someone who wonders if everything is some greater "sign from the Universe" (fact: not *every* single thing is) or my intuition is trying to get my attention because another loved one might be in danger (second fact: trauma and fear clouds intuition), it felt like torture to me. I kept meeting people who had the same illness that my loved one had had, saw posters and billboards advertising medications for the condition, and more. As a distraction while on vacation, I had deliberately picked out several seemingly lighthearted books to take—and it turned out a character in every single book had that same medical condition! I was constantly on edge and further traumatized by all of these things. This is a perfect example of what happens to us in a traumatized state: we become highly attuned to the world around us, perhaps subconsciously scanning for danger, but in the process, we see and get triggered by everyday things we've probably passed by a million times before. I realized that had I been tuned in to any other single thing out in the world, like peaches, I likely would have seen that everywhere. This recognition actually led to a funny mantra I used during that time to keep things light while I did the deeper healing work: *Look for the peaches!* But in all seriousness, what happened as I worked to release the trauma, just like you'll be doing in this chapter, was that I stopped seeing reminders of it. I have to be honest in that this took months of using energy therapy in different ways to overcome the trauma I had experienced, like you'll be learning soon—but it worked. Did all the people with this condition go away? Did all the billboards get taken down? No. The less traumatized I became, the less heightened my sensitivity to it was. This is a perfect example of why it's essential to work with unprocessed experiences.

You already know that emotional memory is stored throughout the entire body. Thanks to the work of Candace Pert, we know that "unexpressed emotions from experiences can get stuck in the body at the level of cellular memory." This is such a simple explanation for why we feel bad when we haven't resolved our past experiences. We are still quite literally *feeling* them. And even if it's at a subtle level, it may only take a "trigger" from that metaphorical glass capsule to awaken it.

While your own unprocessed experiences may not disrupt your life in the way that clinically diagnosed PTSD does, you may relate to what it feels like to have PTSD, when one or a few memories from life takes over all of it. This is, again, why we must deal effectively and consistently with our emotions instead of suppressing them. Otherwise, we are at risk of our emotions becoming part of future unresolved experiences.

Even knowing all of this, there's no need to panic. Again, not all experiences traumatize you. And, not all traumas will need to be dealt with in order to get you feeling better. But the ones that *do* need careful attention. I want you to understand that by working with trauma, we are not trying to force a positive perspective on it or make you be okay with something bad that happened to you. Not at all. What we want to do is release the stress it's causing you, even if that stress is undetected consciously. We don't want these traumas taking up space and energy in your body anymore or triggering you without your knowledge.

Working with unprocessed experiences, as you'll be doing in this chapter, will help empty the metaphorical glass trauma capsule so we stop becoming triggered by the world around us. In other words, you'll be seeing peaches more easily instead of trauma triggers.

But first, let's look at different types of trauma so we can better understand where it originates from.

Types of Trauma

Figuring out what trauma from your past to work on can feel messy or daunting, but we're going to take this one step at a time. First, let's go over examples of common types of trauma so you have a better understanding of what we're dealing with here.

Big "T" Traumas

These are the most obvious types of experiences to recognize because they are so big and life changing. Major traumas include experiences related to injury, accident, violence, abuse and neglect, and more.

Little "t" Traumas

These experiences seem small but can impact you in a big way. They include experiences when you felt ashamed (or shamed), embarrassed, or any other emotion you didn't acknowledge. Little "t" examples could include: a friend turning on you, a parent forgetting about an important event in your life, having to make a hard or life-altering decision, or tripping up in a social setting.

Medical Trauma

This type of trauma is connected to things you experienced in relationship to your health. Many people experiencing chronic illness have medical trauma, meaning that they have unresolved experiences from times when they felt helpless, manipulated, abused, ignored, or misunderstood while seeking help. This can also include a physical trauma like a surgery where there are unresolved emotions (perhaps even just the fact that you had to have surgery) or childbirth experiences. From experience, I also know that merely experiencing illness and all that goes with it—such as friends who don't understand, job loss, and more—can be traumatizing and depressing.

Secondary Trauma

This type of trauma happens when you witness the trauma of another person. This is quite common with caregivers but can also occur if you see a car accident, a fight on the street, or something else as a bystander. Anytime you see another person hurt, secondary trauma can come into play. I see this a lot in my clients who are first responders, such as police officers, firefighters, and health-care professionals.

Grief Trauma

This is my own description of the type of grief that relates to life, because it is such a huge contributor to depression. Grief can even occur during seemingly positive experiences like a move, retiring, or having a baby. Grief trauma can occur any time there is a loss, including a loss of independence, freedom, time, space, or hope. Even the grief over *having* trauma belongs in this category. The grief of not belonging is another one I see quite often. Remember that depression can be the way we grieve over our unmet needs and unfulfilled desires in life, including disconnection to self.

A note about childbirth: While postpartum depression is a medical condition, I have seen that working on grief can make a huge difference. Even the experience of childbirth can cause grief over how it unfolded compared to how we imagined it would be—and new moms and dads often experience grief over the loss of their identity, lost time, body changes, and more.

Collective Trauma

This type of trauma affects groups of people as a whole. Collective trauma is typically linked to historical or cultural events, such as slavery, the 9/11 attacks, war, survivor's guilt, persecution for religious beliefs, racial oppression, and other ongoing events. The COVID-19 pandemic is perhaps the most powerful recent example of collective trauma because of its global effect. In addition, people have had such vastly different perspectives on it, which has opened the door for trauma—not just about the virus itself but about political agendas, inadequacies of our health-care and governmental systems, socioeconomic factors, and more. Collective trauma is difficult enough on its own, but it often also reawakens personal traumas that still reside within us.

Inherited/Absorbed Trauma

This type of trauma occurred before you came to this earth. This kind of trauma can be absorbed while you're in utero, carried in your family lineage and passed down to you, or even come from a past lifetime (there are entire healing systems based solely on resolving these types of trauma). You'll be learning how to deal with this special category of trauma in part IV. As a note: collective trauma can also be inherited, meaning passed from generation to generation.

～～

Now that you understand what types of trauma there are, let's start to figure out what specific experiences you want to work with. Even though there may be a lot, we only need to do one at a time—and we definitely do not have to heal all old traumas in order to feel good. Phew.

A Question to Uncover Unprocessed Experiences

In chapter 10 you are going to learn how to use muscle testing to tap into your subconscious mind and find specific ages and experiences from your past to clear. But for now, a really great way of approaching unprocessed experiences is to use what we know about "the big three" emotions (anger, grief, and fear) to identify unprocessed experiences. While trauma can be connected to any emotion and any experience, the focus on these three is a great place to start because trauma is often closely tied to them. This way of working allows us to continue to deal with those important emotions in the context of that entire web we talked about—wherein emotions, experiences, and beliefs are all tangled up together. In other words, we're kind of getting a two-for-one healing deal here.

By answering the question I'm about to give you, you'll be able to see how "the big three" are relevant to experiences from your past that you haven't yet healed from.

Here's the simple question: *What past experiences am I still grieving over, or angry or fearful about?*

With this question, I urge you to go with whatever events from your past pop into your mind first, *not* what seems most logical. Please ask your brain to stay out of this one because that's how we'll get the best information to work with. And remember, for fear, try to tap into experiences that might have made you afraid to be who—and express who—you really are. When you're focused on this question, try to zoom in on specific experiences that pop up for you, even if they make no sense or seem "silly." I don't often see people with just a single experience driving the depression train, but it's possible there was one incident or experience that was simply the straw that broke the camel's back. If one stands out for you, you'll want to start there. But it's very likely that you'll need to work on a bunch of experiences over time. Every experience you release from your system will help you get closer to reconnecting with yourself.

Here are some additional questions that can spark ideas of experiences from your past to work with: *What still has an emotional charge when I think about it? What images or memories keep running through my mind? What experience was I "never the same" after? What happened in my life in the year or two before I started to feel depressed? What thing from my past do I find myself worrying might happen again?*

Answers to the above questions may include a loved one being diagnosed with a disease, being involved in a car accident, losing a pet, witnessing a tragedy, getting fired from your job, a relationship breakup, being abandoned, caring for a sick relative, being embarrassed in front of a group, being excluded from something, a financial loss, or a health scare.

Hopefully you have a growing list of ideas. Next, we're going to start chipping away at that list.

Some Gentle Warnings

When working with trauma, there are a few things to keep in mind that will help make this the best experience possible for you.

First, and most importantly, while energy therapy tools are easy to use on your own and can be used very safely in this way, please use caution in the case of traumatic experiences or triggering memories. For very sensitive memories, you may need to work with a professional who has extensive training. I don't want you to be scared of doing work on your own, but I also want you to use care and intuition when dealing with trauma. If something feels too scary to talk about or too hard to think about, it's likely not going to be the best thing to work on on your own (especially when you're new to this work). Often, the presence of another person creates a space and sense of security that can make working with old memories much easier and more pleasant. A professional will have the experience and training to make sure you have a positive, healing outcome. If you don't have the means to get that type of support, it can be very helpful to work through this with a friend or trusted loved one. I have many students who pair up with each other, even via the phone, and it works wonderfully.

Next, I hope that through this new understanding about your past you will find compassion for yourself and the trauma (especially what you thought was "no big deal") that might be affecting you today. However, I do not want you to use your new awareness to become a *new* trauma story. Trauma happens because of the human condition, but we should never victimize *ourselves* by making our entire lives about this trauma in ways that are unnecessary. The idea here is to deal with it only in order to move on from it so we can truly leave it behind once and for all.

Finally, and again, even though you likely have a big list, please don't feel overwhelmed or rushed by this process. You just need one experience to start with. You can pick anything on your list, or go with the one you feel most drawn to or charged by. It only takes starting with one to get the "change train" moving in the right direction. We are focused solely on creating momentum in your healing, not rushing to the end result of being healed. We don't have to go from feeling like shit to feeling great all at once. And, in fact, we can't, even if we try.

Now I am going to guide you through some really powerful ways to start this process. Follow me.

Energy Therapy Techniques for Trauma

Together, we'll be working with unprocessed experiences using a combination of Emotional Freedom Technique (EFT) and Thymus Test and Tap (TTT). This is the way we are going to release the trauma from your system and help you truly heal from your past.

Using both techniques gives you two ways into your body in order to release the energy more fully. The cool thing is you already know the basic way to use both techniques.

Let me explain why these techniques together are the perfect combo. Thymus Test and Tap helps us work with the individual stuck emotions within the trauma capsule that we might not have any awareness of. It's one way of addressing part of an unprocessed experience. But it's not complete. Here's why. EFT, which we'll also be using, helps us work with the entire memory, including several aspects of that glass capsule we talked about—not just emotions as in TTT, but images, sounds, details of the experience, and other specifics that might be stuck in your system. Those things can all be "triggering" you, even if they feel like small details. In addition, EFT is a more introspective process, allowing you to work through the actual event while often gaining conscious realizations, cognitive shifts, and emotional understanding and closure that help you move past the experience. Using EFT specifically for trauma has the support of several studies behind it related to its efficacy in this area. This is done very safely and without being re-traumatized by the experience. EFT is used in veterans' programs for PTSD and in hospitals internationally. In fact, I conduct EFT trainings at a major hospital in the New York area for staff and patients to address this very thing.

Thymus Test and Tap (TTT) to Release Individual Emotions

I often like to start with TTT as it's a very gentle way to ease into working with difficult memories. Remember, this technique helps us release the individual emotions that might have gotten stuffed in the trauma capsule without us being aware of them.

THYMUS TEST AND TAP (TTT) UNPROCESSED EMOTIONS	
Section 1	*Section 2*
Abandoned	Helpless
Fearful	Hopeless
Grief-stricken	Heavy
Unloved	Impatient
Intimidated	Out of control
Criticized	Defensive
Judged	Frustrated
Hated	Panicked
Berated	Insecure
Worthless	Powerless
Attacked	Shocked
Betrayed	Failure
Disconnected	Stressed
Section 3	*Section 4*
Rejected	Vulnerable
Angry	Unsupported
Guilty	Undeserving
Resentful	Ashamed
Blamed	Overwhelmed
Indecisiveness	Bullied
Disgusted	Lonely
Conflicted	Alone
Confused	Regretful
Nervous	Disappointed
Unsafe	Discarded
Worried	Excluded
Hurt	Desperate
Resistant	Traumatized

Step 1: Identify an emotion to work with. Sit quietly and ask yourself, *What emotion is stuck from* _____*?* (short description of trauma, for example, "when the doctor told me I was the worst case of depression he'd ever seen and I'd probably never get over it" or "when Bobby beat me up in sixth grade"). Now, close your eyes and very gently swirl your pointer finger all over the list of emotions. You can make big circles or any shape you want, but try to cover the entire list. When you feel called to stop, stop while holding your finger in place. This is your body intuitively picking up on the first emotion you need to release.

Note: If you know muscle testing, you can use it here instead of the finger swirl method. If not, don't worry; you'll be learning how to use it with this technique in chapter 10.

Step 2: Tap your thymus seven times repetitively to release. Now that you have identified the first emotion stuck in your body, you are ready to tap your thymus to let it go. Simply tap at least seven times firmly over your thymus gland with the fingertips of one hand. We are using this tapping to send a force of energy through your system to clear the emotion. I like to say, *Releasing, releasing, releasing* or *Let go, let go, let go* as I tap. But simply breathing as you tap works well too. Tap as many times as you need to feel like you've released it.

Step 3: Take a deep breath and begin again at Step 1. This technique is an excellent way to work with emotions from generational/inherited trauma, collective trauma, or past-life trauma. I give you the protocol for doing this in chapter 11 (it will be easy for you once you get the hang of doing it because it's just a slight variation on this same process).

Note: Remember that with this technique, you may need to repeat it many times to release the related emotions stuck in your body. Just make a note to yourself to keep working on it and you'll get through them. Even releasing a few can make a big difference in how you feel, though.

EFT Tapping for Unprocessed Experiences

To use tapping to release unprocessed experiences, we are going to use the basic protocol for EFT tapping but focus on our feelings about an event from the past versus focusing on how we are feeling now.

I'm going to provide a script to guide you, so all you need to do is tap along and fill in the blanks. I tend to close my eyes, which helps me better focus on the memory than if I'm distracted by my surroundings. Looking at the "picture" of the memory in your mind can really help here. You can even "watch" or imagine it as if it's a movie. Our goal is to "retell" the story as if you were telling a friend, so that we can neutralize it in our bodies and minds.

Note: For working with vague memories or an experience you don't have a lot of detail about, flip to the tapping script in the appendix and look for Subconscious Tapping. That tapping script can/should also be used for very sensitive memories because it allows you to "work around" the details versus diving right into them. Again, remember that if a memory feels very big or scary, it may be beneficial to work on it with a professional. If you feel safe doing it alone, use your intuition in terms of what pace is safe for you.

As a reminder, here are the tapping points for Emotional Freedom Technique.

Emotional Freedom Technique points: Top of the head—*Tapping point:* This is smack dab in the middle of the top of your head. Eyebrow—*Tapping point:* The inside corner of the eye, right where the eyebrow starts. Side of the eye—*Tapping point:* The outer corner of the eye, right on the bone, close to where it meets your temple. Under the eye—*Tapping point:* The top of the cheekbone, right under the eye. Top lip—*Tapping point:* This is where a mustache would be if you had one. Chin—*Tapping point:* In the indentation on your chin, halfway between your bottom lip and the tip of your chin. Collarbone—*Tapping point:* Find where you would tie a tie on your neck, then go out to the side an inch and drop directly under the collarbone. Under the arm/side of the body—*Tapping point:* This is where a bra band is, about four inches under the armpit on the side of the body. Fingertips—*Tapping points:* The lower right-hand corner of each fingernail, where it meets the cuticle. You only need to tap on the fingertips of one hand.

Step 1: Start tapping on the karate-chop point continuously while repeating these statements:

Even though I have this memory of _____ (describe or summarize the picture/scene and what it's about) *and I feel it in my* _____ (describe how it feels in your body, if you feel it there), *I choose to let it go now.*

Even though I feel _____ *about this memory, I choose to let it go now.*

Even though I have this memory stuck in my mind, I choose to let it go now.

Step 2: Cycle through the rest of the points using these statements:

I see _____ (describe the image).

I have this memory stuck in my head.

I feel _____ *in my* _____ (describe the physical feeling you have looking at the memory).

What stands out to me most is _____ (is there a specific part of the picture you're most focused on?).

I don't know how to let it go.

It's making me feel _____ *(hopeless, anxious, etc.).*

I wish I could just let it go.

But I keep thinking about _____.

This memory stuck in my mind of _____.

As always, feel free to revise the script to whatever resonates for you. In the blanks, you want to try to incorporate concrete details from the experience: colors, sounds, smells, the weather, facial expressions, a certain phrase someone said to you that is upsetting, and so on. You can also include intangible concepts or feelings such as feeling discarded, being unable to trust yourself or someone else, someone betraying you, feeling humiliated, and so on.

Step 3: Continue tapping for several more rounds. Tap through all the points while "venting" about what you remember, incorporating any details or thoughts that pop up for you. If you feel any extra "sticky" parts of the memory (meaning they are more vivid, upsetting, etc.), stop and focus on those while you tap until you feel a positive shift. This is essential, as often there are just one or two pieces of a memory that lock the trauma in place, versus the entire experience. Then, once you are feeling more neutral about that piece, continue working with the entire memory. Take a deep breath or two between every few rounds.

Note: I want you to keep tapping until you feel like the memory of your experience is as neutral as it can be, meaning you don't feel much of a charge (*bzzzt*) or you lose "attachment" to the memory in terms of how activated you are by thinking about it. These, along with the memory feeling "far away" or distant, are great signs you are neutralizing it. This doesn't have to happen in a single tapping session. A lot of people tap for a few minutes, don't feel better, and claim tapping doesn't work. But it can take some time. You don't need to completely neutralize the memory before you start to work on another one, but I like to keep a running list in my notebook so I can always pick up on something if I haven't finished. Remember to really talk out the details and tell and retell the entire story of what happened to make sure you are covering all the pieces. It works just like retelling an experience or incident to a friend or family member.

Step 4: Wrap up with positive statements. Once you are happy with the improvement or are done with your tapping session for the time being, do one more round using all positive statements:

I can move forward now.

I can be okay now.

I am safe.

You did it! You officially have a new way of working with trauma that will help you move forward in a totally new way. I hope you found it to be easier, and less scary, than you imagined. I think what you just did—dealing with the beliefs, emotions, and trauma that have been holding you back—is the most difficult part of healing, but you are officially over the hump now. You can now slowly work through the list you've made to let go of unprocessed experiences once and for all. Remember, it's going to help neutralize triggers you might not have even been aware you had. This is true even if you are still experiencing the trauma, such as in the case of chronic illness or pain.

You are now ready to move on to part III of the book to learn how to commit to yourself for lasting change. This is my favorite part.

Create Lasting Change

Addressing Life Patterns

When we come up for air after all we've been buried under, our life may not look the same as when we started. It is now that we must commit to ourselves and create the lasting change we've worked hard for. This means holding ourselves accountable and calling ourselves to our greatness, even if it feels foreign. It's not always easy to commit to ourselves, but it's how the joy finds us.

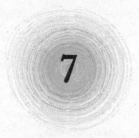

7

Listen to Your Body

As you know, depression can be a wake-up call to help us become attentive to our own needs, at last. Most of us have been ignoring our needs for a long time. And there is nothing—for better or worse—more persistent with communicating what you need to pay attention to more than your body. The spirit is easy to ignore, but the body complains. The body is our best secret keeper and also a truth teller, with its own special language. It communicates with us through symptoms and sensations. These are the body's way of pointing us toward what we need to pay attention to in terms of patterns that are no longer working for us. In other words, it's how the body talks. These symptoms are actually metaphors for what's going on internally, at an emotional and energetic level.

While you should always consult your doctor about any physical symptoms, the phrase "depression hurts" is widely used for good reason. It's a reality for most people. We can't deny that feeling bad emotionally directly affects the physical body.

In this chapter, I'm going to give you insight to help you decode your body's messages in order to help you better understand what you might need to address in your life.

The Body's Hidden Messages

Up until now, we've been working on identifying and clearing emotional energy to heal from depression. But because there is a direct correlation between the physical body and depression, "working backward" by focusing on the physical body can be such an enlightening and productive way to approach things.

Learning your body's language is one of the coolest, most intriguing parts of the feeling-better process, because you begin to understand what has been going on inside of you in a way you haven't up until now. Our bodies are the greatest storytellers of our lives. Our bodies are honest without hesitation. The body often gets a bad rap for interrupting our lives with its needs and missteps, but the body is a mirror for much of what is going on in our hearts. The body will speak and complain until we listen.

I hated my body for much of my life, deeming it a "problem" for causing all the pain and discomfort it did. But in hindsight, I needed this. Because had my body not continued to speak, I would have gone on ignoring so much of what I didn't know I needed to face, and certainly, a lot of what I didn't want to face. The shame is that for many years of my life, I didn't realize my body was my *ally*, not my enemy, talking to me for good reason. Thankfully, it didn't cower in my ignorance or pity me and soften when I resisted listening. It simply kept talking.

Your body is the keeper of the things you might have not noticed, have chosen to ignore (or have tried to ignore), or have been wondering but are unsure about. When you learn to listen to your body and decode its language, you will start to gain clarity about why you've been feeling the way you feel. At the end of this chapter, I will be offering you ideas about exactly how to use your body's wisdom for your healing.

Your Body's Loudest Links

Each person has certain parts of their body that are what I call the "loudest links" (a nicer version of the "weakest link"), meaning they speak louder or more often than other parts. For instance, this can be your back and neck, but for another person it may mean their digestive system. Your loudest links are the places inside you where you tend to hold emotional stress. You may also have certain symptoms that appear over and over, exacerbated at various times in your life. For me, if I become disconnected from my self or allow myself to get too buried under my own "stuff," one of the symptoms I get is body aches. This is my body's unique way of telling me that I am aching for something—more rest, less pressure, or even just lighter expectations on myself. But I have clients who have never had this as a symptom and get migraines instead. These are our body's individual ways of delivering the messages that pertain to each of us.

Once you get the hang of decoding symptoms and sensations, your body's language will become easier and easier to decipher. Then, all there is left to do is listen to what it's saying, either by making a necessary change in your life or by clearing emotional energy related to the message. It is almost unimaginable to me now that I at one time had no communication with my body at all, left totally in the dark and disempowered about what to do for myself to feel better. Discovering my body was talking was a huge turning point in my own healing. This is true for the vast majority of my clients as well. Even though I don't have any major emotional or physical challenges like I once did, I'm still a complete metaphor geek about my own body—decoding even temporary or small issues that pop up for me. If I get a headache, an upset stomach, or feel really tired on any given day, I'm always trying to "read" the messages so that I can work with my body to help resolve the symptoms faster. And over and over again, I've seen with myself and others that this works. This doesn't mean we are denying an actual physical issue or symptom but rather working from the energetic perspective to see if we can help it shift.

An article by Dr. Madhukar H. Trivedi, of the University of Texas Southwest Medical School, reveals fascinating information[1]: Patients who present with a high number of physical symptoms may be more likely to have a mood disorder than patients who present with only a few physical symptoms. Because there is a shared neurochemical pathway with both depression and pain, it makes sense that they should both be addressed for optimum well-being. In additional research described by Trivedi, it was shown that the improvement of physical symptoms corresponds with reduction in depression symptoms. This suggests that when we shift physical symptoms, we may also be shifting the depression. This gives us great motivation in looking at the body's symptoms as a complete approach. This is why I'm insistent on helping you pay attention to your physical body, even though it's likely that your primary issues *seem* to be emotional. Working from both the emotions and the physical body allows us two very different ways "into" your system to help you heal.

How Mind-Body Metaphors Can Help You

Metaphors provide a symbolic way to understand one idea by using another. While the body can't literally speak, it can show us things in ways that we can draw meaning from. I know better than anyone how easy it is to get caught up in physical symptoms, seeking a diagnosis for them, along with a quick fix. But as we all know, sometimes the correct diagnosis doesn't happen and the fix doesn't come. This speaks to the point of how the body's symptoms can mean so much more than just physical malfunction. But even if you do have something physically "wrong" with one of your organs or body parts, I've seen that releasing emotional energy from that area can unburden it and create more "bandwidth" for physical healing.

Releasing emotions in a specific organ, body system, gland, and/or muscle can actually help increase the function of it. The reason is not that emotional healing necessarily "fixes" physical problems but rather that releasing the extra burden of emotions within a system allows that system the capacity and energy to deal with proper functioning (like detox, digestion, and so on). I want to share an example I've seen many times before in order to illustrate what I'm talking about.

I've had a large number of clients who have been referred to me by doctors when nothing else was working to bring down levels of high liver enzymes. As you'll be learning, liver energy is linked to many of your body's functions, such as hormones, digestion, and detoxification. It's also energetically associated with the emotions of anger and frustration. In almost all my cases with these clients, when we've repeatedly released emotional energy from the liver, we've seen that the liver eventually restores proper functioning and that lab tests show healthy enzyme levels again. It sometimes takes a while of working on different angles to see this shift, but again, we are usually doing this when no other modality is working, so let's just say, we have time. The improvement we've seen is likely due to releasing emotional energy that had been burdening the organ energetically and blocking optimal functioning. My work with these clients helped to restore balance to the liver so it could do its job once again. In this example, you can really see how emotions and the physical body are so connected!

Assuming you've already checked with your doctor about any physical symptoms, what will help now is for you to be curious about an alternative (emotional) contributor or hidden meaning behind any physical challenges. This in no way means you caused it; rather, some of the things you've been unaware of have been affecting your whole self.

I don't want to leave out perhaps the most important part of why it's essential to learn what your body is saying: so you can listen. In a lifetime of perhaps ignoring what's going on inside you, listening to your body will help you change that. Listening will help you stay connected to what's going right—and wrong— inside of your body, mind, and spirit. Listening to your body is your guidance system to know when you need to make a change in your life or work through something that's blocking your happiest, healthiest self.

How to Use the Metaphors

This information is not just to notice, it's to utilize. Through symptoms, your body is asking you to release and resolve emotional stress or change something to ease your body in some way. I'll be giving you ways to do that at the end of this chapter.

You already know every body speaks in its own way, but there are some common messages in the way of metaphors I've identified over the years that will be a hugely helpful start for you. The lists I'm going to give you shortly are summaries of my interpretations and ones that have led to healing for many people.

The categories in this chapter are listed in groupings of chakras and then some common conditions related to certain body systems. Because I cannot possibly cover every inch of our expansive, amazing bodies, I've highlighted the main areas that I find most useful for decoding the body's messages. In other words, these are the areas of the body that are often the biggest communicators, trying to tell you what you need to know for a better, happier life. I've also categorized them in the same way my brain does—probably not properly according to the actual science of body systems. So if you are looking where you think it might be obvious in my list but you don't see what you're looking for, check elsewhere.

For each area, I will give you my insight on some of the messages your body might be trying to send you. This is my interpretation through intuition, my understanding of the body's metaphors, the energetic body, and experience in identifying patterns with clients over many years—but please know there are endless options that could be possible for you. You may find that you resonate with several different messages, which is totally normal. Additionally, if you see that similar messages are associated with different parts of the body, know that's normal. Because everything is so interconnected, there are often several parts of the body connected to certain symptoms. What I suggest is exploring all aspects and finding what resonates with you the most.

Some of my interpretations may also spark new ideas for you, which I encourage you to follow. The best thing you can do is stay totally open to this process and whatever your body is trying to say.

If, while trying to figure out your own body's messages, a "random" thought, memory, or image from your life comes up for you, don't ignore it. This is likely related to what your body is trying to tell you or what you need to work with. I suggest that you record in your notebook all the things that resonate with you for the part of the body that's speaking to you. It may be a lot of things, which again, is totally normal. Remember, at the end of the chapter, I will give you a specific protocol for addressing these symptoms and messages from an energetic standpoint. By writing down some ideas as we go along, you may also realize that in some cases, you are being called to make a change or shift in your life to fulfill a need your body or spirit is asking of you.

Chakras

As a reminder, chakras are the spinning energy centers in the body. Chakras store early childhood experiences and old stories throughout the body. Each chakra governs a specific part of the physical body and has a different emotional and energetic correlation. By determining what symptoms you may have located in the area of certain chakras, you can often figure out what message your body is trying to convey. I'm going to help you by giving you some pointers on each chakra and also share common messages of the organs and glands located in that chakra. Because I do not cover every single internal organ, gland, and so on, refer to the main chakra and its meaning if the specific part of body you are feeling symptoms in is not listed on its own.

Crown Chakra (7th Chakra)

The crown chakra extends from the "crown," or top of your head, down to your eyes. It represents your connection to a higher power (to God or the Universe) and is tied to feeling guided, led, and protected. It's also linked to the general feeling of trusting life.

Physical area: Top of the head.

Possible messages: Symptoms that show up here may be general messages from your body about feeling "lost," confused, untrusting of life and the Universe. You might also fear the "unknown" or feel confused or worried over what the next step in your life should be. You may worry you'll never find your way or will be wandering around (and alone) forever.

Brain/head: Metaphors for this area can be feelings of spinning with anger, "fuming," being dizzy with fear, spinning with confusion, feeling so overwhelmed that your "head is going to combust," overthinking, "doing your head in" (by ruminating over the same thing), or being congested with worries. Migraines and headaches are a telltale clue for me that someone is too self-critical or fixated on their mistakes or imperfections. Symptoms in this area can also mean a person has a fear of listening to their own inner voice/intuition. The head is also associated with the liver's energy; and the liver is primarily linked to anger (self-directed or at others), resentment, and frustration—which refers back to being "dizzy with" energy. Dizziness is directly connected to the nervous system energetically, which can be a metaphor for losing your equilibrium or balance because of overwhelm, trauma, and more. Overthinking is also symbolic for head symptoms (think "head spinning," "stuck in your head," and so on).

Third-Eye Chakra (6th Chakra)

The third-eye chakra sits between your eyebrows and is sometimes referred to as the Brow Chakra. It represents intuition, imagination, and seeing your life and self for how they are (interpretation).

Physical area: Eyes, ears, nose, pituitary gland, hypothalamus, skull and frontal lobe of the brain (our emotional center of the brain).

Possible messages: Issues in this chakra may be metaphors for ignoring your own intuition, worrying you don't have any intuition, worrying about the future, being blocked from seeing things clearly, or blocking out what you already know. It's common to feel like you can't "see a way out" when this chakra is speaking through symptoms.

Eyes: Metaphors related to the eyes include not wanting to see or acknowledge the truth, not liking what you see in your life, or being afraid to see something for what it really is. Energetically, the kidneys are linked to the eyes and represent fear, especially fear of "seeing" or "not seeing" something important in your life.

Ears: Physical discomfort or other issues with the ears can be messages about refusing to hear the truth, not listening to yourself, being hurt by what someone else said, and being overly sensitive to hearing criticism or opinions of others. Because the ears are energetically connected to the kidney meridian, and kidneys are associated with fear, it's worth working through any fears you have. Ears can also be linked energetically to the nervous system, which means stress and trauma affect this part of the body (especially with ringing in the ears).

Sinuses: Problems in this area can be linked to being "stuffed up" or "congested" with worry, irritation, and old grief (unreleased tears and snot). The sinuses and stomach are connected energetically, and it's common for people with sinus issues to also have stomach challenges (and vice versa).

Throat Chakra (5th Chakra)

Located in the center of the throat, this chakra is about communication (listening and speaking), expressing yourself, listening to yourself, and speaking your truth. It's also linked to communicating with others. It's one of the most important chakras we have because it's connected to so many important aspects of our lives, primarily our expression.

Physical area: Thyroid, throat, tonsils, mouth, and brain stem.

Possible messages: Problems in this chakra may be general messages about not speaking up for yourself, lack of confidence, not owning your own truth, difficulty expressing your needs, swallowing your emotions, choking back grief or other emotions, feeling like you have to swallow your wants/needs in your life/job, not being or feeling heard, and fear of sharing how you feel or others not liking what "you have to say." It can also be connected to feeling like your voice doesn't matter. For this chakra, it can also be beneficial to work with issues that may be connected to the chakras directly above (Third-Eye) and below (Heart), as I see the throat chakra as the "tunnel" between them. If there is energy stuck in the surrounding chakras, it can block the throat area.

Heart Chakra (4th Chakra)

The heart chakra hovers in the center of your chest. It is linked to love (including self-love), relationships with others, forgiveness, and the ability to bond with others. It also represents your own heart's desires and your ability to manifest them. The heart chakra spins over your thymus gland, the super important gland for the health of your immune system.

Physical area: Heart, thymus gland, lungs, upper rib cage and vertebrae, shoulders, arms, and breasts.

Possible messages: Problems in this chakra can be messages about conflict—especially inner conflict—and feeling "unsettled" in your heart. Symptoms that show up in the chest area (including lungs, chest, and heart) might symbolize your tendency to carry "burdens on your chest," having a heavy heart, fear of opening your heart, feeling like you're being held/pushed back, feeling suffocated (unable to breathe), not being able to catch your breath because life is hard, feeling broken-hearted, and being unable to get things "off of your chest."

Lungs: Energy held in the chest area is heavily linked to grief and not feeling like you have space to grieve, or grieving for losses in your life.

Breasts, specifically: Messages that show up in the breasts indicate that you need to turn inward and nurture yourself and your needs. This might be a message that you are ignoring your own needs, possibly in favor of taking care of everyone else. The stomach meridian, or energy pathway, runs directly through the breasts. Because worry is the emotion most linked to the stomach meridian, incessant worrying (especially about others) can affect the breasts.

Solar Plexus Chakra (3rd Chakra)

The solar plexus chakra sits just below the sternum and governs our sense of personal power and how we relate to and interact with the world. Its energy is tied into self-confidence, self-esteem, and the feeling of being in control of or having power in our lives. It also holds our judgments and opinions about ourselves, and the world.

Physical area: Kidneys, liver, adrenal glands, pancreas, spleen, stomach, gallbladder, and lower rib cage.

Possible messages: Symptoms in this chakra may be general messages about feeling powerless or insecure, and like you don't have a say over your own life. It may be connected to the feeling that you are losing control or having your sense of power taken away.

Digestive system: A lot of your digestive system is covered by this chakra. Problems in this area are connected to not being able to process or digest life and your emotions (especially in terms of letting go with ease, when needed).

Liver/gallbladder: These two organs are specifically connected to things you have the following emotions about: anger, frustration, guilt, resentment, and indecisiveness. Feeling like nothing ever goes right, your life is a struggle, and everyone is out to get you can all be related to the liver. The liver is energetically connected to hormones as well and can affect the endocrine system, so working on any of the liver's energy can be hugely beneficial. The liver is the major detoxification organ in your body, and especially old anger will cause issues here.

Sacral Chakra (2nd Chakra)

The sacral chakra is located in the pelvis behind the belly button. It relates to feelings, joy, creativity, and expression. When those things are repressed, it is directly connected to depression.

This chakra also represents sexuality and governs the energy of self-healing.

Physical area: Reproductive system, bladder, intestines, ileocecal valve (controls and regulates the flow of fecal matter in your body), pelvis, lumbar, and sacrum.

Possible messages: Symptoms in this chakra may be general messages about not allowing oneself to feel joy and holding emotions in (suppression). Basically, if you have issues in this area, your spirit is saying, "You are holding me back." It will be helpful to be honest about the ways you might be doing that in relationships, career, and life in general. Sometimes, it's connected to the message that we feel we need to get permission to be happy or free.

Kidneys: Your kidneys are a big reservoir for your energy and are connected to fear, dread, feeling unsupported, and being conflicted. The kidney meridian runs through your feet and your legs, so fear around moving forward or stepping out on your own may apply. Anything in your life that feels "draining" can be linked to the kidneys and has the ability to affect your entire body.

Bladder: Issues with the bladder are often connected to feeling "on edge" or nervous all the time, and to being "pissed off" or unable to process anger.

Reproductive system: Issues in this system can be offering you messages about resistance—especially to your own expression of joy or creativity in relationship to activities you love (e.g., art, writing, music, dance). Symptoms here might be trying to get you to relax, loosen up, and allow some of your childlike or free-spirited self to be expressed. Fear around creating our lives as we want to or "birthing" a new way of life for ourselves can affect these organs.

Feelings of insecurity (the opposite of feeling secured in the womb) can affect this area. Stuck energy related to sexuality or sexual relationships can also show up here.

Root Chakra (1st Chakra)

The root chakra is located at the base of the spine. It represents your primal energy: instincts to survive and feelings of safety and security. This chakra is connected to basic needs and survival. It deals with the family unit and is linked to feeling grounded or "rooted" in life.

Physical area: Genitals, legs and feet, base of spine.

Possible messages: Challenges in this chakra may be general messages about feeling unsafe and worrying about the future in terms of survival (finances, stability, support from others, etc.). They may be pointing you to messages that you need to heal childhood trauma so you can restore a sense of safety and security in your life. The adrenal glands are connected to this chakra. Adrenal glands are also related to your energy and ability to manage it in a healthy way. Being unable to say no and having fears around disappointing others affect the adrenals. These glands can be suppressed by being "drained" by life.

Knees/back: Weakened adrenal glands can show up as problems with the left knee or low back.

Conditions

Here is a list of different bodily conditions and what the message behind them may be. If you have multiple conditions, take a look at all the messages and see what resonates most. You might find there is quite a bit of crossover.

Chronic Illness

Messages from your body related to chronic illness may be feelings that life is "too much," scary, demanding, or overwhelming—and you feel you don't have a "safe space" to retreat to. It can be linked to metaphorically carrying the pain of your own life and other's lives. Chronic conditions can also be metaphors for feeling like a victim, like life is unfair, and that you are left to deal with all the suffering alone.

Nervous System Conditions

The nervous system is most affected by feeling unsafe and nervous or anxious in life, being suspended in the *freakout* response, always waiting for the other shoe to drop (and believing it's going to happen), and feeling on the "brink of" or "on the edge" all the time. This system is one of the most important to tend to for overall emotional and physical well-being. The nervous system is connected energetically to the bladder, and the bladder is symbolic of being "nervous" (as in a "nervous bladder"). Because being "pissed off" is another message the bladder sometimes sends, it's worth looking at feeling nervous about making others upset, which may affect the nervous system.

Immune System Conditions

The immune system is in charge of keeping you safe and keeping foreign invaders out. Symptoms that show up in this system are often linked to defensiveness and protection: feeling attacked by others or the outside world. If you feel vulnerable and without protection, your immune system may be telling you to work with these feelings.

Autoimmune Conditions

Autoimmune conditions are metaphors for "turning on yourself" or attacking yourself. These conditions are often messages about self-criticism, attacking yourself or your past (regrets), and feeling completely out of control. They can be particularly affected by patterns of carrying guilt or shame, and feeling unworthy or undeserving. They can also be a message that you have self-directed anger you aren't dealing with.

Digestive System Conditions

Imbalances in the stomach and rest of the digestive system are often related to being unable to "digest" life or having time to "digest" one thing before another comes along, being "sick with" worry/guilt/fear, being "gutted" (really upset) and unable to deal with it, having something "eating away" at you, feeling stuck or unable to let go of the old (constipation), feeling "punched in the gut," being unable to metabolize or process something (thoughts, emotions, a situation), or having difficulty "slowing down" your reactions (diarrhea). The lower back is affected by the lower digestive system and the neck muscles are linked to the stomach, so messages might show up in either of these places. The stomach is often associated with the energy of worry, so if you are a worrier, it will often be your neck that delivers that message.

Inflammatory Conditions

While pretty much all conditions have a component of inflammation, conditions that are specifically inflammatory in nature, such as arthritis and irritable bowel syndrome, are often linked to being angry or inflamed, letting old hurts build "heat" in the body, feeling agitated, feeling critical of yourself, not being able to "break down" your emotions but rather holding on to them all, and having a sense of impending fear that causes you to "brace yourself" for life.

Pain-Related Conditions

These types of manifestations are often messages that you have self-punishing patterns like blaming yourself, feeling like you deserve punishment for not being perfect, feeling guilt about the past, or absorbing the pain of others. Pain is a metaphor for the mind and spirit being in pain. People with chronic pain often take everything on themselves, feel responsible for the world, and can't "shake off" the pain of others (are compulsive fixers).

Fatigue-Related Conditions

Fatigue is a message about being drained and not having "enough" for yourself. It can be linked to feeling "tired" of life or "tired" of a specific situation, being without passion, holding heaviness or sadness, feeling exhausted from never saying no, people pleasing, and being overwhelmed and drained from cycles of worry and fear. What we are tired *of* is typically what we are tired *from*. Fatigue can be a metaphor for feeling like "what's the point?" of life and without any energy to deal with things.

Allergies, Sensitivities, and Intolerances

Strong reactions such as allergies are messages about feeling fearful and defensive. The body is misdirecting its fear by trying to protect you from things that are perfectly safe for most people. This is often a whole-body fear response, but it can also be connected to strong emotions you were feeling when exposed to particular substances (e.g., the time you ate macaroni and cheese right after a bad breakup), which then made the body "blame" those foods for the upset and caused a reaction to protect you from them. Working on how fear is "taking over" your life and how you feel it's protecting you will help with calming these misdirected responses.

Sleep-Related Conditions

Insomnia, disrupted sleep, and trouble falling asleep are all related to having an unsettled heart. Sleep challenges are metaphors for internal unresolved conflict in your heart that's preventing you from being able to rest. Allowing others to "invade" your space and disrupt your peace will also show up at night, when our bodies are most vulnerable because of their relaxed state. I always say that whatever you push away during the day will sneak up on you at night because it's the only time we often retreat enough to let it. The more you deal with your feelings in your waking hours, the less they'll come up when you are ready to sleep.

Skin Conditions

Your skin acts as the barrier between you and the world. When symptoms show up on the skin, they can be linked to keeping your emotions "under your skin," feeling like people are getting "under your skin," that you feel unprotected against something or someone, you are "itching" or "burning" to do something or let go of something, and holding hurts right under the surface. Skin rupturing, such as blisters, can be bubbling up agitation. Itching is a metaphor for things you can't fix or "get to." Rashes are sometimes a burst of anger/expression that you've been holding on to, or the body having a "big" or "sensitive" reaction. Your skin is linked energetically to your lungs, which are connected to the primary emotions of grief, sadness, and confusion. The energy of "congestion" can also show up on the skin—feeling congested or stuck with emotion and unable to move it out. I often interpret skin rashes as feeling unsafe and needing to be defensive or protective.

Musculoskeletal Conditions

Because the musculoskeletal system is about support and flexibility, issues here can be metaphors for not being able to move through life with ease, for resisting life's flow, trying to control things, or always pushing against life.

Hands: Problems with the hands can be showing you that you feel you can't handle life or that you try to handle too much.

Legs, knees, hips, and feet: Challenges with the legs and feet can be showing you feelings of fear around moving forward, being ungrounded/unsure of your next step, feeling "stuck in the mud" or too fearful to move, feeling like you're sinking, carrying too much emotional weight, feeling unable to walk away from something, having to walk away from something, and feeling lost/wandering around. Issues with the right knee are often linked to resentment, whereas issues with the left knee are often linked to strained adrenals (tiring yourself out, draining your energy reserves). The legs and feet are connected to kidney energy; so again, patterns around fear should be considered.

Back: Energy affecting your back can be showing you patterns of carrying everything on your back, being unable to "stand up" for yourself, being stabbed in the back, being afraid to "turn your back," turning your back on someone (guilt), turning your back to something scary, living in the past (feeling like it's behind you or following you), wishing you could "go back" and change something, being afraid your past (all that stuff "back there") will catch up with you, being unable to back away from a situation, or having no backbone with others. The lower back (root or 1st chakra) is usually linked to worry about survival, family, safety, and money; the mid-back (solar plexus or 3rd chakra) is often associated with guilt; and the upper back (heart or 4th chakra) may be a metaphor for feeling unsupported or your needs being neglected (especially by yourself).

Neck: Emotional energy showing up in the neck can symbolize being afraid to turn in a new direction, turn away from someone toxic, fear of heading the wrong way, having a "pain in the neck" in your life (usually a person, but it can be something that's dragging you down), afraid to stick your neck out in the world and be yourself, or being inflexible and rigid. The stomach meridian runs through the neck and is associated with the emotion of worry—which means that symptoms in the neck often are related to the stomach.

Now that you have more understanding about what some of your body's messages might be, we need to address them. With these new clues, it's going to be easier than ever to figure out what you need to heal within you.

How to Address Your Body's Messages

There are a few ways to address your body's messages. Perhaps the most important one is to *listen*. If you've discovered that you're being drained by worrying about everyone else, you need to make a conscious effort to change that. If you've realized you're holding on to old anger, you need to make a conscious effort to change that. If you had an epiphany that you are beating up on yourself, you need to make a conscious effort to change that. I'm sure you're seeing a theme here. The point of decoding your body's messages is to listen to them so that you can change your life for the better.

That being said, I know that changing is "easier said than done." We'll first look at how you can use tapping to address the energy that you need to shift.

Tapping

Tapping is a great way to address symptoms and their messages—and to release the related emotional stress you've been holding. The reason tapping is ideal here is because it gives you a way to release stuck emotional energy from your body while also giving you the opportunity to process the issues consciously—which is important for noticing if there are patterns in your life you need to change.

You can use the tapping script below, using any set of points you wish, but remember to start with the karate-chop point.

As a reminder, here are the tapping points for each of the three techniques. Remember, you only need to choose one to work with.

Temple Tapping Points: At your temples on each side. If you only have the physical use of one hand, you can use that hand to tap the temples alternately.

Emotional Freedom Technique points: Top of the head—*Tapping point:* This is smack dab in the middle of the top of your head. Eyebrow—*Tapping point:* The inside corner of the eye, right where the eyebrow starts. Side of the eye—*Tapping point:* The outer corner of the eye, right on the bone, close to where it meets your temple. Under the eye—*Tapping point:* The top of the cheekbone, right under the eye. Top lip—*Tapping point:* This is where a mustache would be if you had one. Chin—*Tapping point:* In the indentation on your chin, halfway between your bottom lip and the tip of your chin. Collarbone—*Tapping point:* Find where you would tie a tie on your neck, then go out to the side an inch and drop directly under the collarbone. Under the arm/side of the body—*Tapping point:* This is where a bra band is, about four inches under the armpit on the side of the body.

Fingertips—*Tapping points:* The lower right-hand corner of each fingernail, where it meets the cuticle. You only need to tap on the fingertips of one hand.

Chakra Tapping Points: Crown (Seventh) Chakra—*Tapping Point:* Top of the head. Third Eye or Brow (Sixth) Chakra—*Tapping Point:* In between the eyebrows. Throat (Fifth) Chakra—*Tapping Point:* Front of the throat. Heart (Fourth) Chakra—*Tapping Point:* In the middle of the chest. Solar Plexus (Third) Chakra—*Tapping Point:* Right under the sternum at your solar plexus. Sacral (Second) Chakra—*Tapping Point:* Just below the belly button. Root (First) Chakra—*Tapping Point:* Top of your thighs (pat them like you're calling a puppy up on your lap).

Step 1: Start tapping on the karate-chop point continuously while saying one or more of these statements three times:

> *Even though my body might be trying to tell me* _____ (describe the message you are working with from the guide I provided above), *I can be okay anyway.*

> *Even though my body might be trying to show me* _____ *through* _____ (symptom or body part), *I can heal it.*

> *Even though my body might be trying to get me to change* _____ (pattern or issue), *I can do that and move forward.*

Step 2: Cycle through the rest of the points using these statements as a guide (add your own or revise mine to feel more natural):

> *I really need to change* _____ (examples: *the way I stress about work, being afraid of change,* or *all this anger inside*).

I must really feel _____ (use the metaphor here: *out of control, like I make too many mistakes, or "tired of" dealing with my ungrateful family*).

I feel it in my _____ (name part of body or body system that's struggling).

I just feel _____.

This hidden message in my body is about _____.

I just feel like I can't _____ (*get the anger out, tell people how I really feel, give myself permission to be happy*).

My _____ (name the body part or system) *must really need me to know* _____ (insert the message).

I think this might be because _____ (what is it connected to?).

I don't know what to do about this but maybe _____ (*release the anger, go with the flow more, decide to meet my own needs*).

I am really struggling with _____ (the topic of the message).

Continue tapping for several more rounds, tapping through all the points and incorporating any ideas or thoughts that pop up. Take a deep breath or two between every few rounds.

Here, you are simply "venting" all your ideas, thoughts, or feelings you have about the message. This can include why this message is true for you, from where in your past the challenge might have originated, and why you might need this symptom in your life, even if just subconsciously.

Step 3: Wrap up with positive statements. Once you are happy with the improvement or are done with your tapping session, do one more round using all positive statements. You can choose any of the following:

I'm releasing this old energy now.

I can be okay now.

I am safe to heal.

This will not likely be a "quick tapping" session, but rather a series of sessions to work through this stuff. By the time you have physical symptoms, the emotional energy has been in your body for a long while. This doesn't mean you can't release it—just that it may take some real open, honest, and intuitive tapping sessions to do so.

Note: Dealing with past trauma can be very helpful if you think about when this message started. For instance, if the message from your body linked to fatigue might be how "tired" you are of how your boss is treating you, it would be so powerful for you to go back and deal with an unprocessed experience you can think of—the time when your boss embarrassed you in front of others or rejected an idea of yours, for example. You can use both EFT and TTT for this, as you learned in the previous chapter.

Thymus Test and Tap (TTT)

In addition to EFT, I recommend TTT to release specific emotions in the particular system or part of the body that is having the symptoms. This helps clear out emotions in relationship to things we might not be aware are connected. This will be a process you do over time, as well.

Step 1: Identify an emotion to work with. Sit quietly and ask yourself, *What emotion is stuck in my* _____ (short description of

THYMUS TEST AND TAP (TTT) UNPROCESSED EMOTIONS	
Section 1	**Section 2**
Abandoned	Helpless
Fearful	Hopeless
Grief-stricken	Heavy
Unloved	Impatient
Intimidated	Out of control
Criticized	Defensive
Judged	Frustrated
Hated	Panicked
Berated	Insecure
Worthless	Powerless
Attacked	Shocked
Betrayed	Failure
Disconnected	Stressed
Section 3	**Section 4**
Rejected	Vulnerable
Angry	Unsupported
Guilty	Undeserving
Resentful	Ashamed
Blamed	Overwhelmed
Indecisiveness	Bullied
Disgusted	Lonely
Conflicted	Alone
Confused	Regretful
Nervous	Disappointed
Unsafe	Discarded
Worried	Excluded
Hurt	Desperate
Resistant	Traumatized

location in the body)? or *What emotion does my body want to release from _____?* Now, close your eyes and very gently swirl your pointer finger all over the list of emotions. You can make big circles or any shape you want, but try to cover the entire list. When you feel called to stop, stop while holding your finger in place. This is your body intuitively picking up on the emotion you need to release.

Step 2: Tap your thymus seven times to release. Now that you have identified the first emotion stuck in your body, you are ready to tap your thymus to let it go. Simply tap at least seven times firmly over your thymus gland with the fingertips of one hand. (If you need a reminder of where you thymus gland is, look back to chapter 3). We are using this tapping to send a force of energy through your system to clear the emotion. You can say *Releasing, releasing, releasing* or *Let go, let go, let go* or just breathe. Tap as many times as you need to feel like you've released it.

Step 3: Take a deep breath and begin again at Step 1.

Now that you know why and how to listen to your body, we're going to make another big and necessary shift in your life: drawing your boundaries. Not having boundaries is a huge pattern that contributes to us getting separated from ourselves, and therefore, depressed. But we're about to change that.

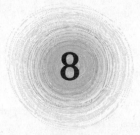

8

Draw Your Boundaries

Boundaries are the protective and invisible parameters that separate you from the world; the distinction between *what's mine* and *what's yours*. Boundaries relate to the ability to say no and consciously choose our involvement in activities, friendships, and what we'll tolerate based on our energy levels, time, and capacity. The thing that I never knew is that having boundaries works with our energy system as a synergistic form of protection. You can't have strong energetic boundaries without the ability to say no—and vice versa.

Boundaries are essential for everyone, yet they are one of the trickiest things to maintain. The real challenge with lacking boundaries is that after a while, it can be almost impossible to distinguish which burdens and responsibilities are ours to carry from which are not.

In this chapter, we're going to talk about how boundaries work, why they are so important, and how to have them.

What Boundaries Are and Why They Matter

Boundaries help you draw a line in the sand to declare: *this* is mine and *that* is yours (or the world's). Having boundaries is the stake of self-care we put down in the ground around ourselves. Reluctance in doing so lends itself to confusion and difficulty in distinguishing who we are, how we really feel, what's ours to actually deal with or feel, and how to effectively be attentive to our own lives and needs. In addition, in the space of not having boundaries, we are sending a message to our bodies and hearts to "let everything in" or take it all on (this is where energetic sensitivity can come into play). Additionally, if we act as if everything is our problem to fix or responsibility to take care of, it can send us into fight, flight, or freeze due to the body's stress response (emergency mode). And being in *freakout* mode may make it harder for us to say no in order to draw healthy boundaries.

I have always been attuned to the needs of those around me— someone who could walk into a room and *feel* it. Even as a child, when I saw an animal or human I thought might be hurting, I hurt too. The pain of others and I had somehow always been one. *I could not soar while others suffer* seemed to be an unspoken pact with myself—a deep-seated agreement from my body that everyone, and everything, was my responsibility. Part of this was certainly being energetically sensitive. But it was not until I was in my thirties that I even recognized the word "boundaries," which should have sounded alarms for my entire life. It was then that I realized not all of my problems could be attributed to energetic sensitivity (as I had thought up to that point), because equally as pervasive was my inability to say a strong and hearty no when I needed and wanted to.

It was only a couple of years ago when I really learned my lesson about boundaries, the hard way (as I admit, I have to learn most things).

While on vacation, I had been emailing back and forth with an organization I was supposed to teach an upcoming workshop for (see: crossed boundaries already, working on vacation). It was a workshop I knew I shouldn't participate in because of some serious reservations I had about the venue that was hosting. Everything in me had been whispering to call it off. I tried, in fact, to wiggle my way out gently, but succumbed.

In the midst of sending and receiving those emails, I was struggling with a "stomach bug." I ended up in the hospital for severe dehydration—turns out that stomach bug was three different strains of E. coli. Yet even on an IV drip from my hospital bed, and with my understanding of how our bodies are affected by stress, I was shooting off email responses, trying to say no—and trying to hold my boundaries without guilt. It is not easy to focus on pleasing others when you are dealing with dehydration, but I was a hero at self-sacrifice. Well-practiced at the art of avoiding hurting people's feelings, I could always tuck away my own wants and needs where they wouldn't bother anyone else.

Just months before this incident, I had read the gloriously written *Year of Yes*, by Shonda Rhimes. Following along on her yearlong experiment of saying yes to the things that scared her most, I rejoiced for her as a reader. But I had an epiphany: for me, saying yes—too often and without regard for my own well-being—was exactly my problem. Much of when I felt depleted or robbed of joy in my life was self-inflicted, easily traced back to my blurred boundaries between *myself* and *other*.

It was only from that hospital bed that I saw clearly—there was never *any* part of me able to distinguish between what was my responsibility and what was not. While much of it felt out of my control because I was empathic, I realized I didn't *always* lack the ability to know what was or wasn't mine to take on. Instead, I lacked the courage to stand up for it. It had never occurred to me before how, if we consciously choose *other* over *self*, our bodies can't know where our own stretched boundaries end and the needs of others begin. When we don't say no, our bodies may say it for us.

My wife once pointed out that all the best things happen to me after I vomit (a bizarre but true occurrence). In fact, she and I met in India following a bout I had with food poisoning. And this issue with the workshop (eventually canceled due to E. coli) turned out to be no exception. Because finally, in my haste, I came to truly "get it," in a way I never had before, that I needed to learn to say no before I *had* to.

It has taken great work on my part to allow myself to be the caring, sensitive human that I am without destroying myself in the process. Still, often, while those around me float through life playing on their phones on the subway or thinking about what to have for dinner, I am sometimes fixated on what needs healing, fixing, helping, *yes*ing. But I have come to learn that when I push myself to say a strong and hearty *no* when I'm able, my body has tended to follow. And it's been worth the work. Because while there may be heroism in saving others, there's also something to be said for the courageous act of relieving your own suffering too.

You're up next.

Yes, You Just Gotta Say No (But Why It's Hard)

No. It's one of the shortest words in the English language, yet the most difficult for many of us to say. No is something that many of us got in trouble for as kids. Stating or demanding our needs is not a popular way to go about the world. It can be perceived as self-centered, selfish, or mean.

People who experience anxiety, depression, and chronic conditions often share the same secret: the habitual pattern of self-sacrifice, suffering for others, or saying yes, even at the expense of our own health and happiness. There is no question that overextending ourselves can have a negative impact on our emotional and physical health.

But saying no is not the simple decision it should be. Let's take a closer look.

Our ingrained programming, survival instinct, fear of being alone or unloved, and habit of people pleasing make *no* a very difficult word for some of us to use. We have been trained since we've been little not to hold our boundaries. It seems like saying no should be such an effortless act, right? But it actually makes a lot of sense why it's not. You're about to see why over-*yes*ing can be such a big part of who we are and how we interact with others.

Childhood Programming

As kids, we look to those around us in order to survive. We learn very early that saying no or that we don't want to do something doesn't get a positive reaction. In fact, we are often punished for it. Don't want to help your little sister? Say you don't want to go to school? It is often considered unacceptable for kids to say no to their parents and other authority figures—and keeping the adults who are responsible for meeting our needs happy is actually a survival mechanism. But when we refrain from saying no as adults, it can really cause trouble.

Fear of Missing Out (FOMO)

The fear of missing out (FOMO) resonates with all of us to some extent, but it is especially common with very social people. In our culture, rest and alone time isn't as popular as "going big" or "living it up." Social media has really amplified the fears we have about being excluded or missing out on things. But it's so essential to turn off these influencers because they are often the reason we say yes when we don't really want to. Something that can help is to think of it as choosing a different *yes* (rest, catching up on chores, focusing on yourself, etc.). At some point, we have to realize that if we push too hard and say yes to everything, we are actually saying no to our own lives and many of the things we really do want to partake in. So it's okay to miss out in favor of your mental and physical health. Saying no feels so good that once you do it a few times, you realize you aren't actually missing that much after all.

Hidden Motivators

We often think of helping as the most selfless act there can be. And while most of the time it's rooted in kindness, often there's another side of the story. "Helping" without regard for our own well-being isn't usually *all* about helping. "Obsessive-helperitis" is a term I use to describe someone who doesn't know when to stop helping, trying, or saving. But this person often has invisible driving motivators that are self-fulfilling (often only subconsciously). You may be thinking, *How in the world is "helping" self-fulfilling?* But helping is so

often a hidden way we feel worthy, control situations to keep ourselves safe (control freaks are the best helpers!), and even distract us
from dealing with our own stuff.

Energetic Sensitivity

We've already learned quite a bit about being an empath, which
may mean you are greatly affected by other people's energy. As
you can imagine, this makes it really hard to feel clear about what's
yours and what's not. Being an empath can indicate our nervous
system is on higher alert than it needs to be, thus being prone to
being in fight, flight, or freeze. While in *freakout* mode, acting from
a healthy place can be difficult, posing a challenge in being able to
say no (and feel safe and good about doing it).

Even though we're going to be doing the deep work of addressing the root of the boundary challenges via energy work, for
now, let's go over some simple and immediate ways to break this
over-*yes*ing (and messing!) behavior.

Questions to Help You Know: Yes or No

The first way to improve boundaries is to understand when to
say no. But if you're used to saying yes all the time, signing up to
volunteer for everything that needs your help, and committing
to things out of guilt, it can be super hard to stop this. You might
simply say yes out of habit. The best way you can break this
pattern is to pause before you say or commit to anything. This will
help you keep your conscious boundary game as strong as possible.
This has taken me a long time to follow consistently, but if you can
do it, too, I know it'll help you so much.

Any small effort you make in the direction of holding your boundaries will greatly benefit how you feel. Even if it's uncomfortable at

first or upsetting to those around you, trust that this will be well worth your effort in helping you to feel better.

Unless it's a medical emergency where a pause to assess might be detrimental, it helps to take a moment to feel into things before jumping in head-first to a *"yes!"* Pausing for a few seconds of time and space to ask yourself the following questions will help you make a conscious assertion about how you are feeling about helping in any given situation.

Will my helping leave me energized, or depleted? This simple question can reveal so much about if this action will detract from your well-being. Some situations may be perfectly beneficial for you. They may leave you feeling good, energized, and fulfilled. Remember, the problem is not deciphering which situations those are, but rather saying yes to everything without thought. Asking yourself how you might feel afterward is a great indicator of if you should participate.

Is it necessary that I get involved? This one is sticky because we all like to feel like we're the only one who can handle something or do it "right." But if something is covered, you may not need to get involved. So much of our energy gets drained simply by trying to control something that doesn't need to be controlled. If there is a group of people working on a project and they are doing just fine, really consider if you have to jump in. Perhaps you do think it would be better if you were there—but is that just you thinking that you'll do it right? Is it the end of the world if something gets done without you, even if not as well? Be careful with this question about necessity, because sometimes our own fear and controlling behavior really get the best of us.

What's my "Why"? Asking yourself *why* you are getting involved can lead to great insight. Sometimes, we're simply saying yes because it's been our automatic go-to response (especially if you are an empath). If you catch yourself being driven by obligation and guilt or a hidden motivator (which usually isn't so hidden once you know what to look for), it's a good indication that saying no is in your best interest. Any answer such as *I have to*, *I should*, *I might regret it* (FOMO), or *I'd be wrong not to* are definitely red flags!

If you still aren't sure what to do, treat your answer as a *no*. You can always change it to yes later. Typically, an "I don't know" is a no from your inner being. But it's much easier to say no from the start versus saying yes and having to backtrack later.

There is no way around the fact that if you want to be able to meet your own needs to be your best-feeling self, you are going to have to learn to say no to things sometimes. But what if this is so new that you have no idea *how* to say it? I'm going to help you with that too.

The Language of No: How to Say It

Even when you decide to say no, it can be hard to know how to actually get it out. It seems easy enough, but if you rarely do it, you might find yourself spending a ton of time and worry on the actual language or way to do it. So I'm doing the hard work for you. Here are my own guidelines for how to say no.

First, say it as soon as you know it. When you decide, reply or communicate your *no* right away. Don't keep your *no* to yourself or it will create time for you to think about, analyze, and talk yourself into feeling bad about your decision.

Next, don't fall into the trap of overexplaining. The more you build around your *no* by adding energy to it, the less clear it is. Simply say no in the most clear and concise way possible to signal to yourself and the other person/people that it's safe and okay for you to be taking care of yourself. Warning: you will have to learn to be okay with any awkward space in conversations this creates—and trust me, it will create some. We get so used to talking and filling spaces with lots of words that when we keep things short, it can feel empty or rude. So we fill them up with excuses and explaining to make it feel better. But it's so much healthier in the long run to be simple and clear. You may even be surprised to find out how easily people accept *no* when you get good at saying it and do so with clear energy. If they don't, though, trust that people will (have to) get over it! It's easy for humans to think that the world revolves around us, but remember that everyone else's world is revolving around them. And even if they don't like your *no*, that's their responsibility, not yours.

You may actually start to see that when you deliver a clear and strong *no*, people respond to it better than you imagined. I've been surprised to find that people often care less than I think they will. And even better, over time, I've come to care less than I used to if they do.

Now, let's go over some language that you can use in your life to make your new habit of saying no a bit easier. These are some of my common responses, and you are most welcome to borrow them! Over time, you might find yourself creating your own too.

Sample Language

The actual saying or typing of *no* is the hardest part. It may take some major bravery, but I know you can do it. Here are some great ways I've learned to say no. I try to always create a positive boundary versus saying no and packing it with a lot of drama and guilt. Your energy really does matter here.

A Simple No

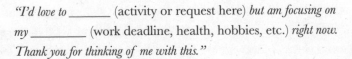

"I'd love to _____ (activity or request here) *but am focusing on my* _____ (work deadline, health, hobbies, etc.) *right now. Thank you for thinking of me with this."*

204

"Thank you so much for the invite but I can't make it. I hope you have a great event!"

"Thank you for asking. I've already committed to something else but I so appreciate you thinking of me." (The "something else" can be napping; it doesn't matter and you don't need to explain.)

"This isn't something I can say yes to now, but please circle back next year/month/week." (Be very cautious with open-ended replies such as this. Only use them if you really do want to do something but can't because of timing or energy levels. For me, I've learned if it's not a *yes* now, it's usually not one later either.)

A Yes with Boundaries

Even if you do end up saying yes to something that feels positive for you, it's still helpful to set limits and healthy boundaries. If you are a person who tends toward self-sacrifice, even a positive situation without boundaries can turn bad. Here are some ideas you can use for setting up boundaries with your *yes*. These set up an expectation for both you and the other person and makes it much easier to stick to what's good for you.

"I'd love to help but I need to leave at 3 p.m."

"This sounds like so much fun, but don't be alarmed if you see me sneak out early. I have a full day the next day" (or *I have a date with myself to catch up on sleep/Netflix/etc.*).

To Fix an Accidental Yes

When you first start to say no more often, know you aren't going to say it quickly and painlessly every time. It might take some serious practice. So if you find yourself saying yes when you meant no, fix it as soon as you realize. Here's some wording for that. The key is to keep it simple.

> *"I apologize for throwing a wrench in things, but I realized I won't be able to _____ (attend, help with, etc.) XYZ* (sub in the event/ meeting) *after all. Thanks again for thinking of/inviting/considering me!"* (A lot of people suggest not to apologize for saying no, but I'm totally okay with it as long as you keep it simple and don't go into overexplaining guilt mode).

Energy Therapy Exercise: Draw Your Boundaries

When we can say no, we have boundaries. Using tapping techniques to work on fears of saying no can be so powerful. We're going to use the following script to release old energy about it being "wrong" or unsafe to say no, so we can do it with much more ease. You can use this script during your energy therapy sessions and whenever you find yourself having a hard time saying no. Eventually you'll have released enough energy that you'll no longer need it. Hooray.

You are free to use any set of tapping points you'd like, but you will start with the karate-chop point no matter what.

As a reminder, here are the tapping points for each of the three techniques. Remember, you only need to choose one to work with.

Temple Tapping Points: At your temples on each side. If you only have the physical use of one hand, you can use that hand to tap the temples alternately.

Emotional Freedom Technique Points: Top of the head—*Tapping point:* This is smack dab in the middle of the top of your head. Eyebrow—*Tapping point:* The inside corner of the eye, right where the eyebrow starts. Side of the eye—*Tapping point:* The outer corner of the eye, right on the bone, close to where it meets your temple. Under the eye—*Tapping point:* The top of the cheek-bone, right under the eye. Top lip—*Tapping point:* This is where a mustache would be if you had one. Chin—*Tapping point:* In the indentation on your chin, halfway between your bottom lip and the tip of your chin. Collarbone—*Tapping point:* Find where you would tie a tie on your neck, then go out to the side an inch and drop directly under the collarbone. Under the arm/side of the body—*Tapping point:* This is where a bra band is, about four inches under the armpit on the side of the body. Fingertips—*Tapping points:* The lower right-hand corner of each fingernail, where it meets the cuticle. You only need to tap on the fingertips of one hand.

Chakra Tapping Points: Crown (Seventh) Chakra—*Tapping Point:* Top of the head. Third Eye or Brow (Sixth) Chakra—*Tapping Point:* In between the eyebrows. Throat (Fifth) Chakra—*Tapping Point:* Front of the throat. Heart (Fourth) Chakra—*Tapping Point:* In the middle of the chest. Solar Plexus (Third) Chakra—*Tapping Point:* Right under the sternum at your solar plexus. Sacral (Second) Chakra—*Tapping Point:* Just below the belly button. Root (First) Chakra—*Tapping Point:* Top of your thighs (pat them like you're calling a puppy up on your lap).

Step 1: Start tapping on the karate-chop point continuously while saying one or more of these statements three times:

> *Even though I have this pattern of saying yes and taking everything on because* _____ *(describe why or include several why's: I'm afraid people will be mad at me; I'll be a bad person if not; I feel*

like it's my responsibility; I'll miss out on something; it feels mean; I can't help it; etc.), I can let it go.

Even though it's so hard for me to say no and when I do it I feel _____ (worried, bad, etc.), I can be okay anyway.

Even though I need to say no, and that feels uncomfortable, I can be okay anyway.

Step 2: Cycle through the rest of the points using these statements as a guide (add your own or revise mine to feel more natural):

I feel like saying no is _____ (scary, wrong, etc.).

I feel like I can't say no because _____ (any idea why you feel this way? Where you learned this?).

I feel this stress around saying no in my _____ (name part of body or body system, if any).

I just feel so resistant.

Part of me is really scared to say no.

What if _____ (people get mad, I'm worthless if I'm not helping people, etc.)?

This old pattern of saying yes—I know it's not good for me because _____.

I don't know how to say no.

I am really struggling with the part where _____ (I have to tell people no, people might be disappointed, I have to let go of control, etc.).

Continue tapping through all the points for several more rounds, incorporating any new ideas or thoughts you have as you tap. Take a deep breath or two between every few rounds. Here, you are simply "venting" about how you feel about saying no, when you say no, and where this might have originated in your past.

Step 3: Wrap up with positive statements. When you are happy with the improvement or are done with your tapping session, do one more round using all positive statements. You can choose any of the following:

I'm letting go of this old pattern now.

I can be okay now.

I am safe even when I say no.

Energy Therapy Exercise: Sweep Old Beliefs Away

You are going to repeat The Sweep script several times in a row while filling in the first blank with what you want to release (the harmful belief). We are going to be releasing these beliefs, one by one:

* "It's wrong to say no/have boundaries."
* "I can only be okay when other people are happy with me."
* "It's my job to take on everyone else's stuff."

Begin the script now:

Even though I have this belief that _____ (state the belief), I acknowledge it's no longer working for me.

I give my subconscious full permission to help me clear it, from all of my cells in all of my body, permanently and completely.

I am now free to thank it for serving me in the past.

I am now free to release all resistances to letting it go.

I am now free to release all ideas that I need this in order to stay safe.

I am now free to release all ideas that I need it for any reason.

I am now free to release all feelings that I don't deserve to release it.

I am now free to release all conscious and subconscious causes for this energy.

I am now free to release all conscious and subconscious reasons for holding on to it.

I am now free to release all harmful patterns, emotions, and memories connected to it.

I am now free to release all generational or past-life energies keeping it stuck.

All of my being is healing and clearing this energy now, including any stress response stored in my cells.

Healing, healing, healing.

Clearing, clearing, clearing.

It is now time to install _____ (permission to say no/have beneficial boundaries now).

Installing, installing, installing. Installing, installing, installing. And so it is done.

As a reminder, you'll want to do this at least three times, or until you learn muscle testing (chapter 10) and are able to check your work to see when you've released it completely.

You are going to feel so much better as your boundaries strengthen! This equates to living your life more for yourself than you maybe ever have, which I'm telling you is probably long overdue.

You are now ready to learn how to commit to your joy by discovering the three promises that will secure the work you've been doing all along. You're doing great.

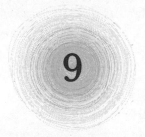

9

Commit to Yourself:
The Three Promises

Sometimes, people do the inner work and are maybe feeling better in some (or lots!) of ways, but are not to where they yet want to be. I feel for them, as I've been this person too. As we talk, I often find a person who has been trying to fix *himself or herself* in order to avoid changing what is no longer working in their lives. The fact is that there's a lot of inner work we can do to help ourselves transform, but it is still our responsibility to actively commit to our ourselves—and our joy.

Much of suffering is self-induced, connected to our inability, and sometimes unwillingness, to simply look at our own bullshit for what it is and say "no more." In this chapter, we are going to learn about what I refer to as "the three promises," which help us call ourselves to our own greatness. As you've learned a lot about so far, old emotional baggage can hold us back. But so too can we hold ourselves back.

Here we are going to talk about why we must not retreat when it comes to our own responsibilities. It is up to us, in the end, to commit to ourselves in a way that draws us toward the most joyful life possible. This is my "tough love" chapter, but you are ready for it.

Promise #1: Tell Yourself the Truth

At twenty-six years old, I was mostly bedridden, my once full life razed back to fit within the soft rectangle of my queen-sized bed: a stack of books I'd never be able to read, bottles of prescription medication that didn't work, quart-size bags of snacks I was too nauseous to eat, and my laptop—the receptacle of my pain when I was able to type into it. It undoubtedly was the worst year of my life, but that's not what I remember as the worst of it. In fact, when I look back upon my life in *worsts* (I know this is a depressing experiment, but stick with me), the details that stand out do not consist of unfavorable circumstances. Every *worst* was rooted in one common denominator: the lie I told myself. And what stands out now are the sad and impressive steps I took to scoot around what I already knew about my life.

If I had any willingness at all to see the truth at that time, I would have seen these things: that the relationship I was in needed to be over, that the career I thought I loved just wasn't what I wanted, and that maybe I didn't know exactly what I needed to make myself happy or healthy, but going through life avoiding my truths had to come to an end. Yet the story I had regurgitated to myself was always: *I'm fine. Everything's fine. Nothing to see here.*

And sometimes, *I don't know* (insert any of the following: *what I want, who I am, what I should do about XYZ*).

So even though at that young age I was closer than anyone ever wants to be to dying, the worst part was definitely not that. It was that I cared more about not further disturbing the already shattered life around me than I cared about my own health—and myself. I saw my own truth as unimportant, a torpedo for the stability in my life I had worked so hard to create. The truth is scary because it disrupts the status quo, which is one of the many ways we convince ourselves of the illusion of safety and control. All those *I'm fines* and *I don't knows* translated deep down under the surface of my terrified being into a consistent, "I know. I know, but I'm too damn scared to let it be true."

Eventually I did get out of the relationship, change the career, and all that—admitting that I wasn't really fine and I did really know what I wanted all along. But it took too long, for sure. And I thought when I did it, I was done forever. But what I know now is that you can't find your truth once and run along on your merry way. Because our truth changes. I had somehow adopted in my life the rule that I wasn't allowed to change my mind, correct course, or start over.

As I have written candidly over the years about my fears and life's atrocities (one of the many joys of being an author), I've become more comfortable with the idea that my truth is a moving target that I must be willing to capture with new curiosity and trust when it arrives. It is one of the primary obligations one has in life.

You have probably heard the saying that the truth will "set you free"? Well, it turns out that's not just an old adage. It's another truth.

The truth is not complicated, although we make it that way whenever we can. It is often scary, still. But what I come back to each time is fact: I am a better writer and teacher, and a happier human when I decide to simply *know what I know* is true.

I think that in your life, you'll find the same. Let's go through it, together.

The Cost of Keeping Secrets from Ourselves

The *truth*—our inner knowing—is something that those of us who are depressed have likely grossly neglected. This is how depression often gets to the point it does. Feelings point to our truth, and truth points to our needs. But sometimes we lie to ourselves to sidestep inconvenient truths; often we wait until we hit a full-on crisis of feeling terrible. Usually we know better than to lie to others. But where we get in trouble is in this lying to ourselves. The simple act of telling ourselves the truth is one of the most difficult things to do. *What if other people don't like our truth?*, we worry. *What if we don't like our truth? Oh my god, what if my entire life gets turned around for WHAT I FEEL OR WANT?* But what if? The cost of not telling yourself the truth is far worse.

Michael Slepian, a management professor at Columbia Business School who studies the link between well-being and secret-keeping, helps us understand why what we keep from ourselves is relevant: a secret in and of itself has no bearing on ill health. This may surprise you as it did me, but this is true no matter what kind of secret it is or how negative the secret keeper perceives it to be. In Slepian's research, the only aspect that had a negative effect was how often the secret keeper thought about or had awareness of the secret and when keeping the secret affected how people felt about themselves. Slepian noted that what did have an effect on health in connection to secret keeping was the "holding back of the real me" part of the equation.[1] This is why what we keep from ourselves can be most damaging—we are essentially splitting ourselves in two, pitting one part of ourselves against the other part that wants to come forth.

Keeping our truth concealed is a masterful way to avoid dealing with our truest and deepest feelings. We sometimes convince ourselves we are fine or don't know what to do or what we want because we aren't in touch with our true emotions. But lying to ourselves is a direct assault on ourselves because we are betraying our own truth—and therefore, our own true selves. Ignoring our truth actually creates a "war" within you, with one part of you having to keep a secret from the other part in order to preserve the secret. This can actually be an act of self-destruction. But we do have good reason to do it.

It is terrifying to show who we really are and what we want. Behind every lie we tell ourselves is an *I'm afraid*. This is why we often get so good at ignoring, suppressing, and talking ourselves out of how we feel, which creates disconnection from ourselves. Who we are consists of all of us: our talents, faults, quirks, and inconsistencies.

In addition, we are trained from a young age to please others. Because from the time we're born we need adults around us to take care of us, we are naturally inclined toward people pleasing. At a young age, it's not necessarily a conscious decision to make others happy, but rather an act of survival. Since telling the truth often gets us in trouble as kids ("I don't like this," "You're mean," "I don't want to go," etc.), we morph into beings that rely on *soft lying* (aka skirting the truth or dancing around it) as a way to stay safe. We fudge the truth about how we feel, what we want, and our true opinions. In fact, especially in the case of families with alcoholism, depression, and other dysfunctions/challenges, kids can become quite the masters at not interrupting the status quo. It's a way we prevent "rocking the boat" in an unstable household.

Over a lifetime of practice, this can easily lead to not being able to easily distinguish the truth anymore, as sometimes we hide things from ourselves that are simply too painful to deal with.

Who we are is at the core of our happiness. When we are not being or living as who we are, there's no way around it— we are going to feel bad. We are literally wired for happiness, with a built-in mechanism that tries to drive us toward well-being. However, we too often force ourselves away from doing what makes us happy because what that is may be an inconvenient truth.

Four Questions to Discover Your Truth

Your truth can be equivalent to your needs. It's at the very core of us: how we interact with life and others around us. The truth has a lot at stake. If we acknowledge our own truth, we may have to make big changes. If we act on our own truth, we may lose the love and support of those around us. And if we show our truth, we may end up unloved. It's no wonder we have such a hard time with this.

I hope you see how and why you could have trained yourself to ignore or become completely cut off from how you feel, what you want, and who you are—for maybe your entire life. But while the consequence of knowing your own truth may feel scary, the risk of not discovering it is feeling like shit.

There is no way you can stay in alignment with yourself without acknowledging what you really want and how you really feel. The problem with having been cut off from it for so long is that we may feel so far from knowing what we really feel and want. But I promise you it's in there and you really do already know.

These questions I have learned to ask help us separate our truth from the fears that block the truth:

Question #1: *If no one else had any opinion about my life, how would I feel?* It's so easy to let what other people think cloud our own clarity. We often value other people's opinions over our own, and sometimes we prefer to listen to others so we're "off the hook" if it doesn't work out perfectly. By filtering out other people's opinions (or even smarter, not asking them in the first place), the voice that speaks to us most loudly about what we should do will always be our own.

Question #2: *If failure wasn't a factor/risk, what would I do, want, or be?* If failure wasn't a factor/risk, we'd all be more aligned with our hearts. The fear of failure and humiliation are very real and very present during decision-making. Equally as important to pay attention to, though, is the fear of success. When we succeed, our lives can change drastically too, and sometimes that's just as scary. Gently looking at our fears is a great way to determine if our indecisiveness is because we're scared to excel, or scared to fail.

Question #3: *If nobody's feelings could get hurt, what would I do, want, or be?* I have always had a major heavy heart about hurting other people's feelings. This, I know, has steered me far from choosing what's best for me, many times. Asking this important question can be one of the most powerful. When we remove our fear of hurting others from the equation, we can usually quickly see what we truly want for ourselves.

Question #4: *If I wasn't trying to be "practical" or responsible, what would I feel or want?* Feeling like we need to be "practical" and "responsible" is often a limiting belief. Of course, we do need to worry about some realities of life, but most times our limits are just created by rules we've been playing by our whole lives. And we never stop to think it might be good to change them. It's okay to stretch our desires into the "fun" and "exciting" instead of the practical, extend beyond the safe boundaries of where we've been living, and know we can dream bigger for ourselves than we've been allowing ourselves to.

In simple terms, all of these questions equate to: *What would my truth be if there was nothing or no one else to worry about?*

There is just no way to follow your own path toward happiness unless you are in touch with *you*. You have to be open to the truth about who you really are, what you really want, and everything in between. This doesn't mean that to feel good, you have to dump your whole life upside down to act on every truth immediately, but it does mean you need to give yourself permission to have your truth.

At some point, though it certainly doesn't need to be now, the decision to make the changes needed to live your life in your truth must come. From where you stand now, to do this fully may feel and be impossible. We have mouths to feed, children to care for, jobs to tend to. It's not always easy to throw your life up in the air to embody your truth, but one must do it as fully as possible.

Are you ready to start? We're going to ease into this by releasing some of that fear you've probably been holding around this—maybe even from yourself—for a long, long time.

Energy Therapy Exercise: Connect to Your Truth

The first step to living your truth is getting comfortable with it. Maybe you are cut off from it, or maybe you have a knowing but can't yet fully embrace it because of fear.

Let's use The Sweep to release some of that old energy that's holding your truth—and all the important information you need for your life—back. Here, we're going to use the The Sweep script to release fears that block us from knowing—or wanting to know— our own truth.

Even though I have this _____ (fear around knowing my own truth), I acknowledge it's no longer working for me.

I give my subconscious full permission to help me clear it, from all of my cells in all of my body, permanently and completely.

I am now free to thank it for serving me in the past.

I am now free to release all resistances to letting it go.

I am now free to release all ideas that I need this in order to stay safe.

I am now free to release all ideas that I need it for any reason.

I am now free to release all feelings that I don't deserve to release it.

I am now free to release all conscious and subconscious causes for this energy.

I am now free to release all conscious and subconscious reasons for holding on to it.

I am now free to release all harmful patterns, emotions, and memories connected to it.

I am now free to release all generational or past-life energies keeping it stuck.

All of my being is healing and clearing this energy now, including any stress response stored in my cells.

Healing, healing, healing.

Clearing, clearing, clearing.

It is now time to install _____ (the belief that it's safe to connect to my own truth now).

*Installing, installing, installing. Installing, installing, installing. And
so it is done.*

Note: As a reminder, you'll want to say the script at least three
times, or until you learn muscle testing (chapter 10) and are able to
check your work to see when you've released it completely.

Promise #2: Lighten the F Up (on Yourself)

My parents raised me with all the love and silliness you'd expect
from the hippies that they were. Both of them always praised me
as smart, sweet, artistic, and kind. But instead of taking these com-
pliments as truth, the part of me that analyzed and internalized
everything contorted them into a rule: *I must be perfect.* With no one
requiring this of me, I took perfection on as my calling, my purpose. As I grew older, the pressure of this undertaking piled on me
like a thousand pounds. I strived to be the one who made everyone
happy and was celebrated for great things, but I also longed to be
one whose faults went unnoticed. When I strayed from the person
I thought I should be—by not getting perfect grades, not being the
perfect friend, or making a mistake—my insides would clench. I
spent a lot of time rehearsing in my head what things I could have
done differently, better. When my parents didn't seem to be both-
ered by any of my imperfections, I worried I might somehow be
less of a shining star to them.

By the time I'd been suffering with chronic illness and my body
had been falling apart for a good long while, I had assigned much

of the blame to myself. Somehow, I must have not done this life thing good enough, perfect enough. Now, perfection was something I owed to the people around me as an apology for being the glaring burden I was. I tried hard to convince myself I deserved mercy in this new small life, yet still, even on my near-deathbed, I felt I wasn't doing sick *perfect enough*.

The truth is this: I was unloved by myself long before anything in my physical body went astray. And it had become painfully obvious that this pattern was crushing my being and assaulting my immune system. At some point, I decided that if I didn't lighten the fuck up, this pattern of perfection was going to kill me. I sensed that maybe it had already started to in some way.

The late spiritual teacher Ram Dass shared what is taught in Tibetan literature: "Embrace your ten thousand horrible demons and your ten thousand beautiful demons." He insisted, "You've just got to take it all and keep going. All your fears have to be embraced, entertained, honored, and you go on with them." And because Ram Dass knew what he was talking about, I decided I would listen.

I began, not easily at first. I had to release all the stories in my head about how my emotions, mistakes, and inconsistencies made me irreparable. I did the work to help myself entertain this new story instead: that maybe no one was keeping score but me. That maybe it was okay to *be* me.

As if adding little bits of elastic at a time to the expectations I set for myself, my life gave way to more leniency, more grace. I laughed at myself more and ridiculed myself less. I made a conscious choice to let go over and over—even and especially in the face of life's hiccups, my own oversights, and the times when "less than" would have never been okay. I decided this was the way I could try crawling toward self-love, or even just self-like. Perhaps I'd make it there in a hundred years, or maybe even a few less. But at least I'd have a chance.

As I practiced, I began to take to the process. I could rest in this new place without the constant pressure. I liked the relief of not always striving for the best and began to affirm that mediocre would fit me just fine. Soon, I enjoyed a delightful side effect to releasing the pressure I had held tight for so long. I began to care a little less about *everything*. I made peace with the fact that not every single decision I made or mistake I made weighed the thousand pounds I was once convinced it did. I found out that being human was so much better than being perfect.

On a recent trip to visit family in stunning Carmel-by-the-Sea, California, with its miniature castle houses and miles of stretched-toward-the-sky cypress trees, I was reminded of the freedom that comes with a life lived by giving fewer fucks.

Carmel is the home of where our favorite people live—including our three nephews and niece. My wife, Charlotte, and I had just said goodbye to two of the kids before flying home to New York. We kissed their sweet cheeks, hugged their sweaty-from-school bodies, and stopped for burritos on our way out of town (because while no one beats New York pizza, burritos are another story). By the time I unwrapped the hot tinfoil, I had become an unexpected mess of tears. Despite my eagerness to get home to our adult lives void of discussions about who pooped when and where, I was heartbroken to leave the kids.

When we arrived at my sister's house to say our final goodbye, our niece Emma's eyes were glossy, the rims of her lids swollen. "I just had a meltdown too," I said. I grabbed her hand and led her up the stairs to her room. "I'll tell you about mine and you tell me about yours." She bit her smile as we scurried upstairs and onto her pale pink bedding, landing on a cloud.

"What happened?" I asked. She shook her head to decline my offer of sharing first. So I did what I've learned to do when someone else is scared: I showed my mess first to prove it would be okay.

"I kept thinking about how sad I was to leave you and I cried into my burrito," I confessed.

Only years before, that same emotional event, leaking out of me at a restaurant, would have caused me to spin into panic, apologizing to all in sight for my flawed responses to life. It would have been a black mark against me in my invisible notebook of *Me v. Perfection*. Two marks maybe, because my wife and the waiter had to see it, too, labeled in my head: CRIED INTO BURRITO BECAUSE I'M A LOSER.

"Did you really cry in your burrito, Mimi?" she asked. "Was it salty after you criiiiied in your burrito?"

"Salt in my burrito!," I swore, throwing up my hand, exploding into laughter.

Emma tilted her head back in a sharp gesture and when it bounced forward again, her mouth was open as wide as could be. This was about the funniest thing she had ever heard.

I really have made it, I thought, Emma and I howling like hyenas. *I may cry in burritos, but I don't care. What a robber of joy I had been to miss out on so many perfect moments like this.*

Lightening up on ourselves does not always come easy, but it's so worth it, and it does come if we let it. In fact, you probably have already done some of this work simply by learning how to be a better conduit instead of criticizer of your emotions. But because I know it's so worth going all the way with this lightening-the-fuck-up plan, I'm going to help you take it to the next level right now.

Where We Start: Less Self-Criticism

It may be that you were born a perfectionist or you grew into one; either way, we've gotta train you out of it. The first thing I do with my clients to help is break this news to them: you are already *not* perfect. You feel better already, right? You're welcome, my friend. You are now already freer than you were even just a few minutes ago. I lovingly throw this fact out because perfectionists are afraid of failing—but it will take some of that pressure off of you to accept that you've already failed in some way. It is entirely impossible to feel good if you are being a jerk to yourself. It just can't happen.

We somehow think that if we push more, are harder on ourselves, or just do things perfectly, we can keep ourselves safe. Loved. But it's all a trap that can make every area of your life miserable.

Self-love. We've all heard this term and been told it will change our lives. But the image conjured by the phrase can feel more like a far-out concept than what it really is. Here's the truth about self-love: it's not about love and light or even thinking everything we do is perfect. In fact, it's kind of the opposite. It's about lightening up about our *imperfections.* Self-love is defined as "regard for one's own happiness." But sometimes, we hinge our happiness on our own judgments of ourselves. So we're going to take another approach here.

You don't need to see yourself as perfect love and light and all the froufrou things that some people insist we feel. But you *do* have to practice being better to yourself. Lighter with yourself. The good news is that I was 100 percent perfect at being hard on myself and have improved by leaps and bounds, so I know how to help you do this too.

Let's just aim for *less self-criticism*, which will lead to less self-hate. This is the best and easiest change we can make to start feeling better about ourselves, even in our human state of lacking perfection. There is no way to heal from being disconnected from yourself if you hate and berate the person you are trying to reconnect to. You cannot bully yourself into doing enough good or being good enough to feel good—and good enough to be loved, especially by yourself. That's just not how it works.

While I promised I'd never force positive thinking on you, what I'm about to ask of you is going to be as close to that as I get. Instead of positive thinking, I want you to practice *lighter thinking* about yourself. This typically comes in the form of self-compassion, but with a little humor. Once we become lighter on ourselves, this lightness tends to reflect naturally on the rest of our lives, in everything we do. Let me show you how it works.

Practice Self-Compassion in Micro Movements

Thanks to Stanford University's Center for Compassion and Altruism Research and Education, we now have scientific data that shows us how and why self-criticism isn't healthy (although we probably didn't need scientific proof on this one). Self-criticism "makes us weaker in the face of failure, more emotional, and less likely to assimilate lessons from our failures."[2] In fact, in a 2012 study published in the US National Library of Medicine National Institutes of Health, a link between self-compassion and negative states such as depression and anxiety was apparent across twenty studies.[3] Because self-compassion is associated with lower levels of self-criticism, and self-criticism is known to be an important predictor of anxiety and depression,[4] this is where we're going to start our work.

Even outside of these samples, there has been much information that's emerged over the years on how positive emotions, including love and acceptance, have a direct impact on your physiology, particularly your nervous system and that *freakout* response we've learned so much about. Because if you are beating yourself up all the time, it makes total sense that your system would read that self-criticism as danger and stress and react to it in just that way.

The practice of self-compassion is learning to lighten up on yourself just as you would with someone close to you who you loved and cared for. You've probably been criticizing yourself for a long time. If this hasn't worked yet, it's probably time to try something new. And this is our work here. You already know the concept of micro movements from chapter 2. We're going to apply those same principles to changing our patterned thinking about ourselves. Here's how: when we have a negative thought about ourselves, we're going to inch our way to the next least shitty thought we can find. Sometimes, and the way it works best for me, is to do it with humor. This is how we inch our way to self-compassion.

For example, if you find yourself thinking, "I screw everything up," see if you can find the next least shitty thing to think about yourself from there. Maybe it will be, "Well, I don't screw *everything* up." And from there, "I only screw up 25 percent of what I do." And from there, "Those are actually not terrible odds." At that, you can stop. If you've been beating yourself up for a long time, then getting to a thought like that is equivalent to a big moment of self-compassion. You did it.

This may seem like a lot of work, but with all the conversations you're already having in your head, you'll see it's not so much trouble at all. Just remember to focus on the goal: the next least shitty thought. In that, you are changing the narrative in your head to be lighter and more forgiving.

Now that you've come so far having released old emotional baggage, I want to point out that you can use this very same approach to start to shift your thinking in all areas of your life. Remember how we decided not even to try to "change our thoughts" because of how the brain processes emotions first? Well, now that you've done such great work in clearing some of that, it will be much, much easier to lighten up your thoughts about everything, little by little. You simply use the "next less shitty thought" response to any negative thoughts you feel would be helpful to shift—about things that happen day to day, your health, relationships, work, and more.

And finally, one last note: give yourself a freakin' break with the big-picture life stuff. One of the most common things people who are depressed tell me is, "If I can only find my purpose . . . then I'll feel better." Our culture is driven by what you do and accomplish in your life. You can't find your purpose in the midst of misery. Because your true purpose is to be happy. Your purpose is to be you. All other secondary purposes come from there. So I'm giving you permission to lighten up here too. Let's get you feeling better first, okay? Then I know you're going to have more clarity about what's next.

Energy Therapy Exercise: Clear the Belief "I Need to Be Perfect"

We're going to use The Sweep script to work with the belief "I need to be perfect." But what will make it more powerful is to come up with a list of whatever comes to mind when we add "because _____" to that belief.

Even though I have this _____ (the belief that I need to be perfect because . . .), *I acknowledge it's no longer working for me.*

I give my subconscious full permission to help me clear it, from all of my cells in all of my body, permanently and completely.

I am now free to thank it for serving me in the past.

I am now free to release all resistances to letting it go.

I am now free to release all ideas that I need this in order to stay safe.

I am now free to release all ideas that I need it for any reason.

I am now free to release all feelings that I don't deserve to release it.

I am now free to release all conscious and subconscious causes for this energy.

I am now free to release all conscious and subconscious reasons for holding on to it.

I am now free to release all harmful patterns, emotions, and memories connected to it.

I am now free to release all generational or past-life energies keeping it stuck.

All of my being is healing and clearing this energy now, including any stress response stored in my cells.

Healing, healing, healing.

Clearing, clearing, clearing.

It is now time to install _____ (the new belief that "I am okay just as I am").

Installing, installing, installing. Installing, installing, installing. And so it is done.

As a reminder, you should complete The Sweep script at least three times, or until you learn muscle testing (chapter 10) and are able to check your work to see when you've shifted it completely.

Promise #3: Take Action

More often than I wish, I will get an email from someone who is in an unhappy marriage or has a life-draining job that is making them physically ill and/or miserable. They pour their heart out to me, listing all the ways in which this situation is slowly killing them, either in body, mind, or spirit. And just as I am ready to reply with the reassurance that within them, they have the quiet courage to save themselves, I see their question at the end: "What energy work should I do for this?"

Years ago, I might have replied gently, with words that I would have wanted myself—something soft. If anyone is sensitive to how hard it is to dump your life upside down, it's me. Because as you'll recall, hard, big choices and changes were once almost as bad as death to me. But what I've learned is this: there is no soft way to approach doing what we need to do to change our lives. There's no choice but to hold ourselves accountable for doing the thing we need to do—when we are able—and to decide our own lives for ourselves. This is where we help you figure out exactly how to go about this with the most ease possible.

The Challenge

While self-healing tools, spirituality, and therapies are intended to support you in your life, I have seen a growing trend where they are used as a crutch to create avoidance of responsibility, action, and change. You cannot meditate, tap, or trust the Universe outta doing what you need to do. I know that it can be the most terrifying thing to even contemplate—making a big shift in your life, especially in a direction that might upset others. But you just can't fix *yourself* in order to avoid making changes in your life when you are able. All the inner work can help, no doubt, especially when it is impossible to change a situation. There is great benefit to feeling better about where you are when you aren't able to change it yet . . . or at all. But it is your responsibility to actively choose the life you want in every possible way you can.

But what if I don't know what to do? you may be thinking. And boy, can I relate. I am a person who used to agonize over every decision at one point in my life, all the way down to the color of my nail polish. Every choice was overwhelming, too much, and felt consequential—as if I was choosing a spouse or a home to buy. The "real" decisions dragged on over years, feeling like half-opened boxes after a move. Everything was undone in my mind, metaphorically labeled "must deal with." In this vein, so much of our suffering is connected to our inability to free ourselves from unnecessary limbo—by deciding to decide. The alternative, inaction, lands us suspended in a state of in-between, living in a state of constant *freakout*, only making change even more difficult.

Even though you may not know what to do quite yet, I hope this work will help you get closer, or find a way to leap sooner.

Resolve Inner Conflict

There are conflicting parts within each of us. Maybe you aren't sure about what to do in a certain situation or what path to take in life. This is so normal. However, if the conflicting parts of us remain in opposition for a long period of time, it can cause great discord—a kind of war within ourselves. This process can drain the energy we need for life, consume our thoughts, and generally make life a miserable game of *What should I do?*

Conflict is typically a struggle between two or more external choices: a yes or no, or choice *A*, *B*, or *C*. Examples of conflicts you may be struggling with include deciding if you should leave a misaligned relationship, changing careers to something you enjoy, figuring out where to relocate, deciding if you should confront a loved one about something, or choosing which medical treatment to pursue. For people who fear making mistakes, even something simple like picking a restaurant for a family meal can become a crippling conflict.

While conflicts with "others" may appear to be an "external" problem, the truth is that all conflict causes a problem within ourselves. Yes, even if another person is involved. Conflict with others often becomes an issue for us because we are *internally* conflicted about how to handle it.

Resolving inner conflict is an essential part of feeling good because inner conflict makes us feel bad. It preoccupies us, puts pressure on us, and creates negative thought loops. Feeling conflicted can hijack your thoughts, causing you to obsess and rehearse scenarios over and over in your mind. In contrast, resolving conflicts sends a clear signal to our body that we are safe to move out of the in-between state.

The Fix: Decide or Make Peace

Almost every conflict can be resolved, to at least some extent, in one of two ways—by deciding to make a decision, or by deciding to make peace with the unchangeable situation. I must add a disclaimer here that if you are in a situation that involves abuse, neglect, or violence, it's imperative to get help. The solution for these situations is not to make peace or "change your energy" or reaction (even though I completely understand that "just leaving" isn't always easy either). We are reserving that approach only for non-life-threatening situations.

However you resolve the conflict, the goal is to make the conflict complete in your head and heart.

The first way to do this is to simply *decide to decide the things that can be decided*. Try to make the swiftest decisions you can. This will cut off the stream of obsessive thoughts about "what to do" because it will be done. This can seem like a scary approach at first—but it works. If you are deciding between a few choices, or a yes or no, decide you're going to make a decision. And do it. Narrow down your options to a small pool. Accept you might never know what's best *for sure*. Then, decide based on the information you have in the moment. And once you decide, get behind that decision like you're 100 percent about it. Go all in. Stop thinking about the alternatives. Don't ask anyone's opinion. People sometimes say to me, "But it's taken so long because I don't know what to decide." And I reply by explaining that if you've been thinking about something for weeks or months (or longer) and you don't know yet, you're unlikely going to just suddenly know with more time. So sometimes, we need to just make the best guess we can and go for it.

You will see that the freedom that comes from moving yourself out of the constant state of inner conflict and limbo will feel so much better than years of being stuck. I'm going to help you in finding clarity for decision-making, but it may also be helpful to review the four questions in the "Tell Yourself the Truth" section of this chapter and see if you can revise them to help you make a choice about your conflict. The coolest thing is that as you make easier choices, deciding becomes so much easier going forward. It will become your new pattern.

The second thing we can do if there is absolutely no choice or decision to be made is to *decide to make peace with the situation at hand*. If we can't change things, we can still work to change our reaction to them. Again, be very selective with this approach, but do use it if there is absolutely no way for you to make a decision. Using this approach will release some of the stress response that's happening inside because you are resisting your current situation and probably feeling like there is no out for you.

Energy Therapy Exercise: Resolve Inner Conflict

We are going to use the Alternate Temple Tapping technique (ATT) to help you resolve inner conflict when there is a decision to be made. I'll share a great process that works for bringing about clarity—often making decision-making a whole lot easier.

Alternate Temple Tapping: To Help You Decide

ATT is perfect for resolving an inner "war" because it's directly linked to the triple warmer meridian's *freakout* response. When we tap to release the yes/no or this/that conflict, we are coming out of being stuck in order to move forward.

Step 1: Start tapping on the karate-chop point continuously while repeating these statements:

Even though I am so conflicted about _____ (describe the inner conflict), *I am open to deciding*

Even though I feel _____ (explain why you feel torn and about what), *I choose to find clarity.*

Even though I am so unsure about _____ (describe the inner conflict) *because* _____ (why is this decision so difficult?), *I can be okay anyway.*

Step 2: Tap alternately on the temple points using these statements as a guide (add your own or revise mine to feel more natural):

I feel so conflicted.

I keep worrying about what if _____.

What if I do the wrong thing?

I feel so torn.

I don't know what to do.

I just keep thinking _____.

I feel _____.

It feels like no decision will be perfect.

I am really struggling with _____.

Continue tapping for several more rounds, tapping through all the points while "venting" about how you feel. Incorporate any ideas or thoughts that pop up during your practice, and take a deep breath or two between every few rounds. This process is equivalent to clearing the windshield on your car on a foggy day. It often results in better clarity and a calmer way to move through things.

Remember, you are simply "venting" about this inner conflict and what you're torn about. This means anything you feel will work. It can be anything you think or feel about it. No one else will ever know what you say or think.

Step 3: Wrap up with positive statements. Once you are happy with the improvement or are done with your tapping session, do one more round using all positive statements. You can choose any of the following:

I'm releasing this conflict now.

I can decide and move forward now.

I am safe.

Alternate Temple Tapping: To Help You Find Peace with What-Is

Because ATT is so powerful in resolving that inner tug o'war, it can help even when you're not able to make a decision—so that you can become at peace with what-is by feeling differently about it. The interesting thing is that once we release energy around this, we are often able to see solutions we didn't before.

Step 1: Start tapping on the karate-chop point continuously while repeating these statements:

Even though I hate that I can't just _____ (describe what you want to do or would do if you could), *I can be okay anyway.*

Even though I feel _____ (explain how you feel about not being able to make this choice), *I can be okay anyway.*

Even though I can't resolve this conflict in my life, I can find a way to feel inner peace anyway.

Step 2: Tap alternately on the temple points using these statements as a guide (add your own or revise mine to feel more natural):

I feel so trapped.

I just wish I could _____.

This is so unfair.

I am so stuck and can't see a way out.

I can't do anything.

I just keep thinking that _____ (life is unfair, no one else has to deal with this, etc.).

I feel _____.

It feels like I'll never find a way out.

I am really struggling with _____.

Continue tapping for several more rounds, tapping through all the points while "venting" about how you feel. Incorporate any ideas or thoughts that pop up during your practice, and take a deep breath or two between every few rounds. You are just "venting" here about all the things you feel regarding not being able to change whatever you are wanting to change. This means talking about how this makes you feel, what you'd change if you could, and maybe why it seems so unfair.

Step 3: Wrap up with positive statements. Once you are happy with the improvement or are done with your tapping session, do one more round using all positive statements. You can choose any of the following:

I can be okay no matter what.

I can feel peace now.

I am safe.

You have now successfully journeyed through your mind, body, and spirit, and done the most important thing you will ever do for yourself—pay attention to your own life. While it may have felt daunting and impossible at first, you persevered. Your commitment and micro steps have, I hope, led back to yourself in many ways, or at least gotten you that much closer than you were before. While it's now time for us to move into learning next-level approaches for when you're ready, there are a few words I'd like to share here first.

And Here We Are, Still

For me, the final conversations I have with my readers toward the close of every book are the trickiest to get just right. All along, I always write each word to you as if you are my friend. But for this book, it was even more so. This book has been my greatest challenge: a privilege, but also an insurmountable amount of pressure. I couldn't put my finger on *why* as I struggled with the format (*How will you learn the best?*), content (*What do you really need to know?*), and style (*How can I make such a heavy topic lighter?*). But I see it now.

I know the deep pain that depression can cause, not only individually but for an entire family and beyond. My dad's depression changed the kid I was. My own experiences with depression changed the adult I am. But I can say without a doubt, from here on the other side, it's so often from these kinds of struggles that the best version of ourselves is born. And this happens not in spite of our pain, but in part because of it. Perhaps it couldn't be so for my own dad for reasons I will never know. I do often wonder, *What if he'd had these tools?* But I am thankful that with this work, so many others have lived out a different story. And my struggle with this book has been simply to make sure I've helped you to feel that it is possible for you too.

In Mary Oliver's famous poem "The Summer Day," she asks of us, *What is it you plan to do with your one wild and precious life?* While the question can feel overwhelming to ponder, I hope that your reaction to it is not that.

I hope that after our time together and the work you've done and continue to do, you now see things in a different light. I hope you have lightened up on yourself and dropped some of the shit that has dragged you down. I hope, mostly, that you will keep feeling. Keep healing. And that you will go and live your one wild life, even and especially if it means sometimes saying no, finding your own quiet joy that no one understands, and giving a few less fucks than you ever have before.

You deserve it, just *because*.

PART IV

Next-Level Approaches

Moving Forward

You have arrived. Take a deep breath. When you're ready to keep going, keep going. Here, we're going even further into your own unique specific challenges—and therefore, your healing.

10

Get Answers from Your Subconscious Mind: Muscle Testing

While the "figuring out" part of feeling bad can be torturous, I'm about to teach you something that's going to make that aspect so much easier. Throughout this book, I've guided you to releasing energy related to the most common types of experiences, beliefs, emotions, and patterns that contribute to depression. But now, it's time for you to learn how to identify even more that will help you heal.

You already know that your subconscious mind holds information about everything in your life, right? This means that it also holds information about exactly what you can do to move yourself forward.

With a technique called muscle testing (also called *energy testing* or *applied kinesiology*), I'm going to teach you how to identify very specific information in your own subconscious mind that is going to unlock a new world of healing. By tapping into your subconscious mind—which has all the information from your entire life—you are about to become privy to some awesome data that you've never had before. This was an absolute game-changer for my own healing, and I trust that it will be for yours too.

In this chapter, you'll learn how to use muscle testing to tap right into your subconscious mind and get endless access to the well of information locked in there, so you can target energy therapy even more precisely than you have been until now.

How Hidden Information in the Subconscious Will Help You

Remember that the subconscious mind is like a human computer and has records of all of the experiences of our lives, including memories, messages, feelings, perceptions, and events in our lives. You can only imagine how helpful this information would be if you only had it to use, right? As I mentioned, I've been leading you through the most common core issues related to depression to put a giant dent in the volcano of "stuff" you've been releasing. But now, I'm going to teach you how to find out exactly *which* experiences from your past are having the most impact on you, specifically *where* in your body trauma is being held and *what* beliefs are holding you back the most. I'll also help you with how to use muscle testing to make the techniques you already know even more effective for you.

If you've been feeling a bit like you've been fumbling through the dark until this point, this chapter is going to turn the lights on for you.

The process of identifying exactly what's in your subconscious mind will help you become even more empowered to release or change it. We have been working with the subconscious mind in so many ways, but now we can—for lack of a better term—get *into* it by actually communicating directly to ask for exactly the information we need.

For example, you've probably cleared some important memories related to trauma. Anytime you clear trauma, you are benefiting your body by calming your *freakout* response, thus enabling your body's own healing mechanism. However, you may have connected some of those memories to depression by using logic or guessing. This is totally fine, but it is possible that not all of them are actually the ones most closely linked to feeling bad. Maybe you remember a particular experience from your life, such as when you were fired from a job just a month before the depression started. And while an event like that could surely be a contributing factor, that memory might feel like one to work with only because it makes sense to your logical mind. Fired = depressed. Seems legit. By following that lead, you could use the logical angle of *being angry or sad from being fired contributed to depression.* And you could totally be right! But because emotions are not always logical, it could instead be linked to another (or other), less obvious event from your past.

While the brain will always try to solve a challenge in the most logical way, sometimes this healing process is a little bit of the Wild West! Intuitively, though, we do know what we're doing. I always say, the body heals in its own order and by its own process. The problem is that we don't usually trust it or go along with it easily. We're now going to focus our work on what I see makes the biggest difference the most often, which is addressing emotional energy that leaves us saying, *Really? That is connected? I'd never have guessed!*

This is exactly why, now that you've worked with a lot of things, including the patterns I guided you to from my years of experience—the perfect way to start—it's time for an additional, yet totally different, approach. This new way of working will help you get even closer to the root of what's been going on with you. Let's learn about muscle testing and exactly how it works.

Muscle Testing

Muscle testing is super cool because it will allow you to identify and release emotional blocks and patterns that you've probably never even thought of before. By doing so, you open yourself up to results you've never gotten before. Muscle testing will essentially direct you to exactly what to do next . . . and after that . . . and after that. I've been using muscle testing for about ten years now and have seen that my own intuition has grown exponentially in that time. I used to be one of those people who insisted I had no intuition. When I tried to tap into it, as suggested by others, I got nothing. Zero. Zilch. But now I'm one of the most intuitive people I know, and I even have the ability to identify intuitive information for others in just seconds without any thought or effort. I credit muscle testing for a lot of this, because it acts as training wheels for intuition. It helps open up new pathways of communication between the mind and body.

As I've used muscle testing over the years, the information I've found in my subconscious was often seemingly ridiculous, sometimes mind-blowing, and kind of embarrassing. But this is why I love it! It's given me insight into what I lovingly call the "crazy part" of me that I don't have regular access to (which may be a good thing). Muscle testing helped me make huge healing progress because of all the new ways I started seeing the challenges in my life.

Muscle testing originated in the early twentieth century as a way to measure the strength of muscles of people with polio. Over a decade later, George Goodheart, a chiropractic doctor, developed a new way of using muscle testing, called applied kinesiology. By applying a little bit of pressure to muscles, he was able to detect weaknesses and imbalances in the body's meridians, which (as you know) are part of your energy system. Testing a patient's muscles is done routinely by physicians as part of a standard neurological exam. Have you ever had the doctor test your reflexes or how you're able to resist a small amount of pressure when they push against your arm or leg? It may seem like they are testing the power of your muscles and your ability to push back when they push. However, because muscles are related to nervous-system function, what they are testing is the health of the muscle when they deliberately "stress" your nervous system slightly. Hang onto that concept because it's all going to make sense in a minute. Applied kinesiology, as it became known after Dr. Goodheart's discovery, is an extended version of the basic exam that your doctor does.

As you've learned, the body is energy—its own sort of electrical system. This system interacts with our physical body and our subconscious mind. The nervous system is closely tied into this dynamic, picking up on the world around us, including very subtle energetic frequencies from our environment. This electrical (or energy) system, which is connected to our subconscious mind, is influenced by all energies, positive and negative. You'll remember from when we learned about the energy system that if something has a negative influence on our electrical system and does not help maintain or enhance our body's energy flow, the energy system will temporarily "short-circuit," affecting the flow of energy going through muscles, glands, and other organs. Well, this short-circuit temporarily weakens our muscles too.

In order to find out what our subconscious mind and body are in agreement or resonance with, we can use the principles of the strength/weakness muscle test. By asking the subconscious mind questions directly and "testing" our muscles' responses to those questions, we can interpret what our body's answers to those questions are. Muscle testing is a super cool way to directly communicate with your subconscious, as if you have a telephone line to it (at last!). This is a sophisticated technique to support and extend the work you did in chapter 7 ("Listen to Your Body") to figure out what emotional energy is blocking your connection to yourself so that you can fix it. Muscle testing will add even more clarity to your healing process. Let's walk through exactly how muscle testing will work in terms of our purposes:

* If we ask a question or make a statement that our body and subconscious mind *agree with* at a core level (meaning the statement is true for us), our electrical system will continue flowing without a hitch and our muscles will retain their full strength. It will be clear to you that you are keeping your strength in relationship to the statement/question.

* If we ask a question or make a statement that our body and subconscious mind *disagree with* at a core level (meaning the statement is not true for us), our energy system will temporarily short-circuit and our muscles will quickly weaken or lock up. You will be able to feel this reaction in the way of some muscle "give." This temporary state is not dangerous at all but allows us to determine what is "weakening" our system (the false presumption, in this case).

You can use the basic process I just outlined in terms of muscle strength or weakness to detect or identify the emotional blocks that are weakening or stressing your system and need to be cleared.

These muscle responses open us up to a pretty clear language with our bodies—a way to interpret what the body is saying without much guessing. The only part you have to figure out, which we'll get to soon, is what questions to ask. But I'm going to help you there.

Muscle testing is an *energy detection technique* as opposed to an energy therapy technique like the ones you've been learning. Muscle testing and energy therapy techniques work together in the same way that the conscious and subconscious minds do. You can heal by using just one or the other, but together, you have the fullest healing power behind you. Muscle testing is the tool that will let us identify what energetic blocks exist so we can point or target the techniques in an even better way than before.

Now, let's learn how to do this thing.

Different Ways to Muscle Test

There are many muscle-testing techniques out there, but I'm going to show you just a couple that I really like. The key to muscle testing is not to get too caught up in the mechanics of it, but rather to be curious and relaxed as you go through it. Don't worry about doing it perfectly. We are using this tool as an alternative to using logic or guessing. And while I find muscle testing to be very accurate, we are just utilizing it to find out information to fine-tune our work, so our lives don't depend on you getting right or wrong answers. In fact, you should never, ever use muscle testing as a substitute for diagnostic testing, your intuition, or a professional opinion. We'll go over those rules in more detail later, but for now, don't put pressure on yourself during the process. We're simply trying to dig out some more clues to help you feel better. All the information we get is a bonus to the great work we've already been doing.

While muscle testing is quite simple, not everyone does it with success instantly. In fact, it took me quite a while to "get it" and a year to really master it. But I really think some of that had to do with me not following my own rule: no pressure allowed. It truly is so important to relax, detach from what the answer might be, and focus only on the question or statement. Because your body responds to the energy of thoughts, emotions, and more, if you are thinking about what the answer will be, what answers do or don't make sense, and so on, it will interfere with the answer. I totally understand the desire to analyze (I'm a Virgo, after all!), but for this tool to be useful, you need to be relaxed. Remember, this is a really awesome tool to have, but it's not necessary in order to have success with my approach. So be light about it.

I'm going to show you two ways to muscle test—the Standing Test and the Hook Finger Test.

The Standing Test

The *Standing Test* is a great beginner's muscle-testing technique that a lot of people like. Let's talk about how it works. Using your body as a pendulum, we are going to see how you respond in relationship to certain statements or questions. Because your nervous system affects your motor response (movement of your body), we're going to be gauging these movements to get our answers. Your body will naturally be drawn toward something that it resonates with or agrees with (your "boss"—aka your subconscious mind) and will naturally be repelled by something that it doesn't read as the truth for you (again, via your subconscious mind).

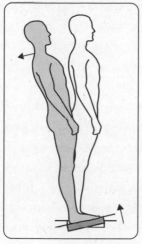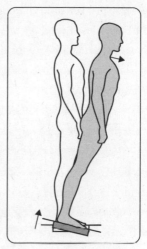

"No" or Not True Response   "Yes" or True Response

Standing Test

Now, here's the trick. We are not muscle testing for fact. We are muscle testing to see what your body agrees or disagrees with. The reason this distinction is important is because we are simply trying to find out what's true for *your* body in order to help you change it if it's not conducive to you feeling good. For instance, we know that if your body-mind believes you don't deserve to heal, you're going to have a hard time healing. So if muscle testing indicated you are holding a belief like that, we'd want to change it. We are using this technique to find out what's true in the subconscious mind (based on your beliefs, experiences, and resonances), not what's necessarily *true* in the world.

If you ask questions when your body is in a natural, standing, relaxed position (but is still able to move without obstruction), it will involuntarily sway—either slightly backward or slightly forward—which will help you determine if it is aligned with something or not.

Remember, words are just energy, so using them will create some kind of response in the body. Your involuntary response will be to move toward (forward) for the truth or reject (push away from) something that's not true for you. Don't worry, this will be a gentle pull. You won't fall over.

If you aren't able to stand, the Standing Test can be performed in a chair—as long as you can sit up in a relaxed position without any back support. Here's how to do it: Stand or sit up straight, with your feet in a natural stance, about shoulder width apart. Make sure your toes are pointing forward. It helps if your shoes are off during this process. Relax your body, with your hands hanging down at your sides. If you have good balance, close your eyes just to eliminate distractions and take a big deep breath.

You are now ready to ask your body for information. Your energy system will be picking up on the energy of what you are saying and reacting to the questions involuntarily. You don't need to do anything but relax so your body can sway easily.

Your body is typically going to sway forward for a "yes" response and backward when it's saying "no." However, I have some clients who have varied responses that don't fit in this box. For example, some lean to the left for "yes" and stay still for "no." Or, they lean to the right for a "yes" and left and back for a "no." The exact movement depends on your body's own unique response. It's not wrong at all. We can still "read" the answers accurately as long as we've decoded how a specific body shows us those answers. So be open to your body's own language too.

First, let's do a baseline test. This is just to see how your body does with this so we can trust the rest of the testing as accurate (remember, the accuracy is not life or death, but it is nice to know the effort is worth it). Say this statement out loud: *Show me a yes.*

Your body will involuntarily tip—probably slightly forward—meaning "yes." This is an indication that this is true for *your* body-mind. Think of this as a head nod for "yes," but with your whole body. Next, say this statement out loud: *Show me a no.* Your body will involuntarily tip—probably slightly backward—meaning "no." It is showing you that it is rejecting or is repelled by what you're saying. Remember, variations are totally fine.

If you are not moving or are getting totally weird responses that you can't figure out, it's most likely because you are dehydrated or your energy is a bit off. No biggie. Drink some water and even tap on your thymus gland for a minute or so to reset yourself. Also, relax, relax, relax. Being too cerebral or controlling interferes with the body's ability to sway naturally in response to the questions. Just keep trying. I'm also going to be teaching you a second technique, the Hook Finger Test, in case this one just isn't quite right for you.

Let's try using this technique now to get an idea of how helpful it can be. Say this statement out loud and notice your body's response: *I have an unprocessed experience contributing to depression.* Alternatively, you can ask it in question form: *Do I have an unprocessed experience contributing to depression?* Whether you use a statement or question format doesn't matter at all, so do whichever you prefer.

Now, relax and let your body sway naturally and tip either forward or backward. This swaying is how it will give you your answer. This will happen without you consciously doing anything, so if you try to "help" or predict the answer, it will interfere with the accuracy. If your body leans forward slightly, your subconscious mind and body are essentially saying, "Yes, I'm in agreement with what you just said." This means that at a core level your body resonates with having an unprocessed experience stressing your body. This is all at a deep, subconscious level. This is a very typical response, even if you've cleared a bunch of experiences already. So don't panic. This is exactly why muscle testing is helpful. I'm going to be showing you later all the types of questions you can ask.

Let me show you the other muscle-testing technique now, as you may prefer one over the other.

Hook Finger Test

I really like this alternative to the Standing Test because it can be done a little more quickly and is also inconspicuous, which means you can use it with more versatility. I call this the *Hook Finger Test*. With your nondominant hand, make a loose fist and position your hand so the top of your hand is facing up toward the ceiling. Now, stick your pointer finger out and make a "hook" shape (like a fishing hook) with it, with the tip of your finger pointing down. I'm going to call this the "hook" finger from here on out. You are going to be using this "hook" finger as your *testing* muscle and the pointer finger of your other hand as the *tester* finger.

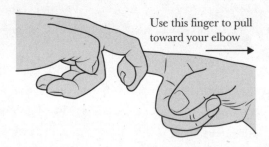

Use this finger to pull toward your elbow

Hook Finger Test

Just like you did with the Standing Test, you're going to either formulate a "yes" or "no" statement or ask your body a "yes" or "no" question. After you make a statement or ask a question, you'll use the pointer finger of your dominant hand and hook it onto the "hook" finger of your nondominant hand. If you're looking at both hands, your two pointer fingers will be hooked together—the tip of your dominant pointer finger will be facing toward you. You will then gently pull with your testing finger (dominate side) toward your elbow to see if the hook finger (nondominant) stays strong under pressure or wants to "open" up or buckle under the pressure and weaken. If the answer from your body is a "yes," your hook finger will easily stay in hook formation against the pulling gesture of your other finger. If it's a "no," you'll feel your hook finger weaken and want to open under the pressure.

Now, with enough strength, you could surely open the hook finger if you tried hard enough. But that's not the point of the technique. We are instead trying to gauge the muscle response: Is it easy to keep it hooked, or does it lose strength? Muscle testing is not a fight of strength between your fingers. You are simply noticing if the hook finger weakens with the slight-to-medium pulling pressure from your other finger. It may take some playing around with to get the right calibration, like getting the flame on a gas stove just right. With practice, you'll figure out a way that works for you. You could also try using other fingers in the same manner to see if that works better for you. Or try touching the tip of your hook finger to your thumb on the same hand to create a circle; then use the finger on the other hand to try to break the circle open while gently pulling.

Answer Key for Muscle Testing

Here is a quick key you can refer back to especially as you first learn to use muscle testing.

The Standing Test

Forward sway = "Yes, I agree."

Backward sway = "No, I don't agree."

The Hook Finger Test

Hook finger stays strong (or "hooked") under pressure = "Yes, I agree."

Hook finger straightens under pressure = "No, I don't agree."

I can't emphasize enough the value of muscle testing, but I also want to remind you that it can take some time to be able to use. In fact, I first learned muscle testing in a group class with dozens of people, and I was the only one who couldn't do it at first! Thankfully, I didn't give up and kept using the healing work without it—and eventually it just clicked for me.

Muscle Testing FAQ

Because I've been using and teaching muscle testing for so long, I typically get asked the same questions over and over. I'm sharing my answers here in the hope that they'll be helpful for you as you learn.

Help! My body is giving me mixed signals. What can I do? First, make sure you're not dehydrated. Electricity requires water, and if you're dehydrated, your energy system won't be flowing like it should.

Make sure you aren't overanalyzing. Relax. Move to another spot in the room. Move away from electronics (for example, take that cell phone out of your pocket). Face another direction. Take a few deep breaths. Try again.

Try to ask the question or say the statement in a different way. Be clear and concise. The shorter, the better. Sometimes the body won't respond if we're not on the right track, or our question needs to be tweaked slightly. Try to change the way you ask the question, just as you would adjust how you said something to a child who didn't understand what you were saying the first time.

Pause between questions and let yourself recalibrate. Going too fast will lead to sensory overload, and your system could scramble your energy, yielding confusing answers.

Use only affirmative language. For example, if you are trying to find out if you believe deep down that you *can* heal, use the statement *I can heal* and see how your body responds, instead of using *I can't heal.* It can be confusing to the body to use negatives in this way while muscle testing.

Why can't I use muscle testing for everything, such as to determine if I'm pregnant, have a certain medical condition, or get the winning lottery numbers? Muscle testing should be used as a tool only to see what your body is in *resonance* with as far as energetic blocks, so you can change and release emotional energies that are no longer working for you. Your body doesn't know what lottery numbers will be chosen. As far as determining physical conditions, it's never a good idea. Naturopaths, integrative practitioners, and chiropractors often use forms of muscle testing to detect imbalances in the energy system of a patient and to find remedies to resolve them, but this is a totally different ballgame than what I'm teaching you here. When you muscle test, you are simply looking for strength and weakness in a muscle, not searching for facts. I and many other very proficient muscle testers can tell you from experience that using this tool in the wrong way will only lead to confusion and misery.

I don't believe the body responds to medical terminology. The programming in your subconscious mind has recorded experiences, perceptions, and more—but it isn't a doctor.

How can I trust my subconscious if my subconscious might be sabotaging me? You can trust your subconscious to give you accurate answers for what your body is in resonance with. This is exactly what we're testing for, and your subconscious will provide it because we aren't asking for opinions or universal truths. We are only asking for what it is or is not in resonance with.

How do I know I'm not influencing the answers? I used to worry about this, but I have found that this really isn't an issue. I kid around that even my teenage clients get answers via muscle testing that they wouldn't necessarily want. And if a teenager can't rig the system, no one can! But honestly, because most of the time we don't actually care what the answer is (since we are using the answer for information only to help us), the conscious mind has no good reason to try to influence the answer. It would be like cheating at a game you are playing with only yourself.

Note: If you are having trouble with muscle testing, I've provided some ideas that will help in chapter 11.

Check Your Work with Muscle Testing

You can use muscle testing to check if you've completely cleared whatever energy you are working to release. This is so helpful when you are wondering if you've really addressed any issue to its fullest extent. Here are a few examples of how to do this.

Unprocessed Experiences

Let's say you are working with an unprocessed experience and are not yet sure if it's neutralized. You can check with muscle testing by asking: *Is this* _____ (name of experience) *still contributing to depression or causing stress on my body?* If you get a "no," the coast is clear. If you get a "yes," simply keep working with it to make sure you are releasing all of the details, concepts, and feelings that come up for you. As I noted in chapter 3, when you first learned the energy therapy techniques, sometimes we need time to "process" the work we've done. So if you've done all you can on a certain subject and you are getting a "no" to it being completely resolved right after using a technique, it's okay to leave it alone and come back to check on it later. It may be easier after a break to assess if there's more work to do.

Beliefs

If you are working with a belief, simply state the same belief after you've done your clearing and muscle test to see if it's still true for you. If it is, you will need to repeat the exercise as many times as needed until it's released.

If a certain energy you are working with is not clearing and you don't know what to do, try layering techniques (using more than one to get total resolution of an issue). I'll show you how to do that in the next chapter.

Use Muscle Testing to Choose a Technique

Once you've worked with all the techniques in the book, you can actually learn to use each one for multiple purposes. For instance, I've taught you how to use The Sweep to clear beliefs. However, you can actually adapt it to help clear *any* type of energy or address any issue. (I'll be giving you lots of ideas on how to do that in the next chapter, with a guide to how to use techniques in a versatile manner.) You can also use muscle testing to tap into your body's wisdom about which technique would be most beneficial and efficient in helping you address whatever you're working on.

To do this, you can ask the following question: *Would it be most beneficial to clear* _____ (insert a short description of whatever you're clearing, such as "the belief that I'm not good enough") *using* _____? (state the name of any technique). Depending on which technique your body chooses, you can adapt the technique to address the issue. Again, I'll offer specific ideas for this in the next chapter. Alternatively, you can use the finger swirl method that I originally described when I taught you the Thymus Test and Tap technique in chapter 3. To do that, you'll write all the techniques on a piece of paper. Then, close your eyes and swirl your finger around the page to see which technique your body is drawn to.

Muscle Test to Determine How Long to Use Each Technique

In addition to using muscle testing to determine *which technique* to use, I use it regularly as a general guide to determine *how long to use a given technique*. You will still want to check your work afterward to make sure it's cleared, but this gives you an indication of where to start. Here are some examples:

The Sweep

Ask with muscle testing: *Do I need to use The Sweep* _____ (number of times) *to clear this belief completely?* If you get a "no," ask again, using another number. And so on. Don't be alarmed if you get to six or more times. Sometimes this happens! Personally, I once had to do The Sweep over a hundred times to clear something completely (but a number like this is very, very rare). Thank goodness you don't need to do them all in a row.

Tapping

Ask with muscle testing: *Would approximately* _____ (number of minutes) *of tapping be sufficient?* Start with about five minutes and work your way up. As you clear and process, you'll want to recheck periodically as things change. If you get a really high number, like sixty minutes, don't panic. This will likely decrease as you work on it. Also, you definitely do not need to do all the minutes in one sitting. You can break up the sessions.

Use Muscle Testing for the Thymus Test and Tap Technique

When you learned the Thymus Test and Tap technique, I showed you how to identify emotions in the chart by swirling your finger over the words on the list. However, you can very effectively use muscle testing for this too. In fact, it's my preferred method to use with this technique. However, it can be considered advanced, which is why you're now ready to learn it.

To find the emotions, I use a process of elimination to find the one my body is looking for. Let me show you how. First, get into muscle-testing position, then ask your body: *Is there an emotion stuck in my body that would be beneficial to release now?* You can change the wording to whatever you want. It doesn't have to be exactly as I've suggested above. I sometimes instead ask, *Is there an emotion that my body wants to let go of?*

Next, ask: *Is it in section 1 (of the list)?* If you get a "no," you'll know it's in one of the other sections and can ask about each of them until you get a "yes."

Once you get to the correct section, I recommend splitting the list in half visually within that section, asking, *Is it in the top half?* (There is no definitive top or bottom half in each section, but I just kind of gauge it with my eyes.) If it's in the top half, you know to focus there. If it's not, you know it's the bottom half of the list within that section.

Once you have the general idea of where the emotion is located, read each word on the list, one by one, asking your body, *Is it _____?* until you get a "yes."

You'll release that emotion as you normally do and then start this process over to find the next one.

Muscle Test to Identify Specific Unprocessed Experiences from Your Past

As you might have experienced in chapter 6 when we worked on trauma, figuring out which experiences from your past are unprocessed can be a little tricky. But using muscle testing is an amazing way to figure out which experiences would be most beneficial to work on—and even which ones are affecting you most.

I love using muscle testing because we can start from scratch (aka knowing nothing) and end up with a concrete and valuable experience to work with. Muscle testing also allows you to be objective in identifying experiences from your past versus using logic. You get to just ask your subconscious mind which experiences are contributing to depression. And because it already knows the answers, you're that much closer to working on something super relevant that will help you feel better.

To muscle test for unprocessed experiences, simply ask your body: *Do I have an unprocessed experience contributing to _____?* You can fill in the blank with: *stress in my body* or *feeling depressed* or *feeling miserable*, or whatever you'd like. I do suggest playing around with a few ways to ask. The answer will most likely be "yes." Even though I've done so much work over the years, I can still find things to clear if I try. Remember that any one person has lots of these types of experiences, but it only takes working with one at a time to get you moving in the right direction.

Next, you can discover through muscle testing at what age this event occurred. Ask: *Did this event occur between the ages of 0–20? 21–30?* And so on. Keep asking until your body answers "yes" to a specific time frame, and then ask about each year within that time frame to get the exact one. You can even ask if this happened in utero, if it's a generational energy, a past-life energy, and so on (in the next chapter, you'll learn how to address these). If you get that the event happened at age 0, that means it was at or around birth.

When you've gotten the age, simply stay open and allow ideas to come to you. Remember, it can be anything, from an obvious experience like a relationship breakup, to something you might consider minor. Just go with whatever comes up. If you are unsure, just keep asking questions, such as, *Was this experience related to _____?* (a person, your career, health, etc.). It's really a big guessing game!

Your body will keep answering you, and eventually, you will probably remember the experience, or simply have enough information to work with. Even just knowing, for example, that there is an experience from age ten that had something to do with your dad will be enough if you can't remember more. There is a tapping script in the appendix for dealing with this exact scenario. You can still clear the energy even if you never figure out what it's about. Such a relief!

Once you think you know what the experience is, it's smart to double-check it via muscle testing just in case your logical brain is taking over here. Ask: *Would it be beneficial to clear_____* (describe it briefly)? Remember, you can also use your own wording.

Once you get your confirmation, you have something to work with that you now *know* is linked to feeling bad. Remember, if you can't identify or recall the specific experience, you can definitely clear it with only as much information as you could collect via the question-and-muscle-test process. Let me give you another example to really drive home my point here. Maybe you end up with the information that something happened at age twenty and it was linked to your job at the accounting firm, but you can't quite figure out anything else. That's totally enough. Usually the body will allow us to release it (even if we only have a few details) if we approach it the right way. Again, you'll be learning how to do this shortly.

Now comes the fun part. In the next chapter, you'll find more ideas about how to use the techniques you already know in new ways. Plus, you'll learn advanced protocols to build upon what you've been doing already.

The next chapter is where you become the true master of your own healing.

11

A Healing Guide: Protocols to Address Specific Challenges

You've now learned so much about depression and how to work with your energy system in relationship to it. In this chapter, I want to show you everything together so you can see it in big-picture format. I'll also be showing you how to clear some specific challenges, as promised throughout the book.

As a reminder, using my energetic approach, healing from depression comes from the following:

* Releasing the "stuff" (aka emotional baggage) that's been blocking you

* Reconnecting to your true self—who you really are

* Living a life of attention to your own needs

We've been doing so much throughout this book to work toward these together. Now, I'm going to share more for your continued journey.

I've put together this guide full of great things you can chip away at. They are organized into three sections: by *specific challenge*, by *chapter and topic*, and by *technique*. There's no need to follow the order in which I present these ideas to you or go in any specific order of which energies to address. And please remember, you don't have to fix it all, or all at once (or, you know this by now, and not all perfectly). Simply pick and choose what resonates for you and follow your intuition and impulses. You can use your skill of muscle testing to determine what's most beneficial to start with or just randomly pick and start somewhere. It all gets you to the same place.

If you are comfortable with muscle testing, I always recommend testing these ideas for yourself, and then once you've addressed them, checking your work to see if there's more to do.

Finally, at the close of this chapter, I'll be giving you some simple ideas about how you can build your own energy therapy sessions to work within.

Specific Challenges

Some of the most common challenges pertaining to depression are nightmares, difficulty sleeping, invisible triggers, energetic sensitivity, and postpartum challenges. Here's how I handle them.

Disturbed Sleep

Nightmares are common and such a disruptive part of life that can terrorize you day and night—even though they occur only when you sleep. Because of my own extensive experience with nightmares, I have a great protocol for working with them. But this approach will often work for any type of disturbed sleep. I've had the most success working with sleep issues within the paradigm of the *threat stimulation theory*, founded by Antti Revonsuo, a Finnish cognitive neuroscientist and psychologist. The threat stimulation theory is based on the concept that nightmares are a way we practice surviving in threatening situations—being chased, falling, violent acts, and more. While we think of our dreams as contributing to an unstable emotional state, it's actually quite the opposite. Our emotional state is what kicks off our dreams.

Here are a few great ways to work with nightmares or other sleep disturbances such as restlessness or constantly waking up by jolt. Each technique typically requires some persistence. Even knowing all I do, I once had nightmares for about six weeks straight before all the emotional work took hold and they dissipated. So keep at it.

* Use TTT to clear "emotions triggering nightmares/ sleep disturbances" (you may need to do this daily for a while).

* Use tapping (ATT, EFT, CT, or a combination) to clear the need for this threat stimulation (use the tapping script in the appendix as a guide).

* Use The Sweep to clear the belief *I need to practice saving myself/protecting/preparing myself in my dreams*.

Other Sleep Difficulties

Trouble falling or staying asleep is one of the most common problems I see in our overstimulating, stress-prone world. But you can work on it with energy therapy, which can make a huge difference. Difficulty sleeping typically has to do with "matters of the heart" (conflict) and feeling unsafe at a core level. Here are a few ideas of how to handle this issue:

✳ Use TTT to clear "emotions preventing restful sleep" (you may need to do this daily for a while).

✳ Use tapping (ATT, EFT, CT, or a combination) to clear energy about worries or fears that might be coming up at night while your "guard" is down.

✳ Use The Sweep to clear the belief *I'm unsafe when I relax.*

Invisible Triggers

Invisible triggers are things we don't realize are causing us challenges. However, if you look at your life's patterns, and even how you feel day to day and hour to hour, you can often start to identify triggers. If you have one in mind and aren't sure, you can muscle test and ask, *Is _____ a depression/stress trigger for me?*

Let's go over protocols for the most common invisible triggers. By doing this, you will become familiar with the format you can use to work with other invisible triggers you may identify.

Note: In the section "Guide by Chapter and Topic," immediately following this section, you will also find many ideas (see "Deal with Your Feelings")—because many of the things I cover there can also be triggers.

Times of day/night: Times of day/night (that is, within a 24-hour period) can be a big trigger. This can happen when you have a subconscious association with something negative from the past and a specific time of day or something general like "the dark" or "the night." For example, I had a very hard time in the

mornings at one point in my life before realizing it was around
the same time that my dad had died many years before. The
energy around the trauma of that time of day had gotten stuck in
my body, but once I worked to clear energy around it, my mornings got much better.

* Use muscle testing to determine what time (or times) of day
  are negatively affecting you.

* Use tapping (ATT, EFT, CT, or a combination) to clear any
  unprocessed experiences linked to that time of day.

* Use The Sweep to clear the belief *I'm unsafe at* _____
  (time of day, or *in the mornings*, etc.).

* Use TTT to release emotions getting triggered around that
  time of day.

People: Certain people may trigger us, even if what we're
triggered about has nothing to do with that person. For example, someone's voice can remind us of something traumatic.
Or someone who asks for our help can trigger us because of
our difficulty in holding boundaries. Here are some ways to
work with that:

* Use muscle testing to determine who is triggering you (it
  may even be loved ones who are very positive in your life!).

* Use TTT to release emotions being triggered by _____ .

* Use tapping (ATT, EFT, CT, or a combination) to release
  old experiences this person reminds you about.

* Use tapping to clear energy related to a person that this
  person reminds you of in a negative way (simply talk and
  tap about whatever comes to mind).

Specifically for empaths:

❊ Use TTT to release emotions absorbed from others.

❊ Use The Sweep to clear *the energy I absorbed from others that no longer serves me.*

Foods/smells/substances: We can have all kinds of reactions to our environment. I see these as energetic allergies: the body overreacts to something in an effort to protect you. This often comes from the link between having felt strong emotion or experienced trauma at the same time as you were exposed to this food, smell, or substance. I've seen miraculous results working with clients by working with their energy system in terms of reactions. But please be cautious, as energy work does not take the place of medical care.

❊ Use tapping (ATT, EFT, CT, or a combination) to release your negative reaction to these substances (use the tapping script in the appendix as a guide).

❊ Use TTT to release emotions associated with _____ (whatever you're reacting to).

❊ Use The Sweep for the belief _____ (insert name of food/smell/substance) *is dangerous for me and I have to overreact to it in order to keep myself safe.*

Seasons/temperatures/weather: Seasonal affective disorder (SAD) is a very real issue that many people struggle with. And while it's not exactly the same as invisible triggers, the success I've seen in people shifting this reaction comes from using a similar protocol. Although SAD is typically an issue during the darkest winter months, some people have a similar issue in the summer or even during the shoulder seasons. In addition, reactions to weather—for example, rainy days or windstorms—and even reactions to humidity can be worked on using the following techniques:

* Use TTT to release emotions linked to _____ (temperature, season, etc.).

* Use tapping (ATT, EFT, CT, or a combination) to release any unprocessed experiences that your body may be holding on to linked to past seasons.

* Use The Sweep to clear the belief _____ (insert whatever season, temperature, or weather affects you) *is dangerous for me.*

Energetic Sensitivity

Here are some guidelines for working with energetic sensitivity, meaning you are overly attuned and affected by the emotions of those around you:

* Use TTT to release emotions contributing to energetic sensitivity.

* Use tapping (ATT, EFT, CT, or a combination) to work with how you feel when you are around others.

* Use The Sweep to clear the belief *I can't relax or be happy while other people suffer.*

* Use The Sweep to clear *this old pattern of taking on other people's stuff.*

Postpartum Depression

While postpartum depression is a medical condition, my clients and I have used energy work successfully to help shift it. Here are some guidelines:

* Use TTT to release emotions contributing to postpartum depression.

❋ Use TTT to clear emotions stuck in the body from labor and birth.

❋ Use Tapping (ATT, EFT, CT, or a combination) to work with how you feel, including any fears, guilt, grief, or resentment about being a parent.

❋ Use The Sweep to clear *energy contributing to postpartum depression*.

❋ Use The Sweep to clear *energy contributing to* _____ (insert any specific fears or other challenges related to being a parent).

Guide by Chapter and Topic

We've worked a lot on different emotional energies: being stuck in *freakout* mode, dealing with feelings, clearing harmful beliefs, healing trauma (unprocessed experiences), listening to the body's messages, holding boundaries, and removing obstacles to help us commit to our joy. Here are some more ideas to continue releasing energy in each of those areas.

Getting Unstuck (Chapter 2)

As you know, calming the nervous system and its *freakout* response is no easy feat. But you've already done so much to make headway in that area. Here's more to work with:

❋ Use TTT to release emotions triggering your "fight, flight, or freeze" reaction.

❋ Use The Sweep to clear "causes for this *freakout* mode in my body."

❋ Use tapping (ATT, EFT, CT, or a combination) to release energy around "feeling/being on edge" (use the tapping script in the appendix as a guide).

Clear Harmful Beliefs (Chapter 4)

Almost everyone who feels depressed has some subconscious block to healing from it. But beliefs can be any stressful ideas about the world. They are all important to clear (but, thankfully, it's not necessary to clear all of them).

Make a list of reasons why your subconscious mind might believe you need depression. Ask this powerful question: *If my brain had some crazy idea of why I shouldn't feel good, what would it be?* If you're able, use muscle testing to confirm which beliefs are true for you at a core level. (If you can't confirm, clear them anyway to cover all your bases.)

* Use tapping (ATT, EFT, CT, or a combination) to clear specific unprocessed experiences from the past where you might have gotten the beliefs you now have. When you identify a belief, see if you can figure out what unprocessed experience it originated from (hint: what past experience might have taught you what you now believe?).

* Use TTT to clear emotions that are causing you to hold onto depression.

Deal with Your Feelings (Chapter 5)

Dealing with your feelings is one of the most important things you can do for your well-being. Here are more ways to deal with them, including clearing out stuck emotions from the past. Emotions stuck from your past can actually be triggers of their own, which is another great way to work with your past.

* Use TTT to release stuck emotions. Muscle test and ask, *Can I release an emotion linked to _____?* Insert any of the following:

   ◦ Energy in a specific part of the body (it's helpful to address the area where you feel symptoms, if any)

- ∘ A specific person (*Mom, Dad*, etc.)

- ∘ A time period in your life (*high school, my first job*, etc.)

- ∘ A specific job (*when I worked at* _____)

- ∘ A theme (such as *intimate relationships* or *difficulty finding jobs*)

- ∘ A fear you have (such as *a fear of flying*)

- ∘ A pattern that's hard for you to break (*self-sabotage, being critical*, etc.)

- ∘ A specific place (such as *my childhood home*)

- ∘ A symptom (*digestive issues, migraines*, etc.)

- ∘ A specific age (*age ten, age thirty-seven*, etc.)

* Use tapping (ATT, EFT, CT, or a combination) to work with however you feel or just tap using *I don't even know how I feel!*

* Use The Sweep to clear *this feeling of* _____ *(anger, hatred, sadness)*.

Heal Trauma from the Past (Chapter 6)

Clearing unprocessed experiences can make a huge difference for you. You can even clear them if you can't remember all the details.

* Use tapping (any tapping technique, but EFT is typically the best choice for traumatic experiences) to clear unprocessed experiences (particularly events that occurred before the onset of the depression).

* Use TTT to release stuck emotions related to those specific experiences.

* Ask via muscle testing, *Would it be beneficial to clear a stuck emotion from* _____ (state the experience)?

274

❋ Use The Sweep to release *all old energy from* _____ (state the experience) and install *I can now move on from* _____ (state the experience).

Advanced Protocol: Inherited, In Utero, Collective, and Past-Life Trauma

All of these energies can contribute to depression. There has been extensive study and work in all of these fields, but here's a starting point to working with these energies.

First, you'll muscle test to see if there's a type of energy you can work on. Simply ask your body using muscle testing: *Do I have an inherited/in utero/collective/past-life (generational) experience causing stress in my body or contributing to depression?* If you get a "yes," you can use the same process as you did for getting more information about unprocessed experiences from this lifetime (chapter 6).

❋ If you get a "yes" for inherited, you can ask your body which side of your ancestry it came from—mother or father? If you want, you can think back to experiences you know your ancestors went through and see if you can locate the person who it was passed from, and the experience itself.

❋ If you get a "yes" for in utero, you can figure out when it was by asking if it occurred in month one, two, and so on, of the pregnancy.

❋ If you get a "yes" for collective, you can figure out what event caused it.

❋ If you get a "yes" for past life, you can ask your body how many lifetimes ago this was.

To clear all of these types of energies, you'll use the same techniques you learned to use for your own, but tweak things just a bit.

* Use TTT to clear emotions linked to *inherited/ in utero/collective/past-life energies* (do them each separately).

* Use The Sweep to clear *all energy no longer mine to carry, especially from* _____ (insert experience if you know what it is).

* Use tapping (ATT, EFT, CT, or a combination) to release whatever you know about the experience or energy (use the Subconscious Tapping script in the appendix as a guide).

Trauma from Specific Ages/Years

Sometimes, we have a very difficult age from our past in which we endured stress or trauma—or have a year or two, where because of our age, it was difficult to process stress—and that energy gets stuck with us. In fact, this type of energy is often triggered in parents when their own child hits around that age. Here are some ideas for addressing this type of energy:

* Use muscle testing to identify ages to clear (you can also test by year, such as 1986, 1987, etc.).

* Use TTT to clear emotions stuck from that age/year.

* Use The Sweep to clear *old energy from* _____ (age/year) *that's still affecting me negatively*.

* Use tapping (ATT, EFT, CT, or a combination) to work with unprocessed experiences from that age/year.

Listen to Your Body (Chapter 7)

Your body's messages and metaphors are giant windows into what you may be struggling with on an emotional level. Here are some ways to address those messages to find relief and peace:

* Use TTT to release stuck emotions related to those specific parts of the body.

* Use The Sweep to release *all old energy from* _____ (state unprocessed experience that you think might be linked to the symptom's message) and install *I can move on now*.

* Use The Sweep to release *the fear of* _____ (state a fear you think you might have linked to your body's messages).

* Use tapping (ATT, EFT, CT, or a combination) to talk about your body's message, why it might be there, where it might have come from, and whatever else comes to mind.

Draw Your Boundaries (Chapter 8)

You now understand how important boundaries are to protect your emotional well-being. Here are some great ways to work on strengthening them even further:

* Use tapping (ATT, EFT, CT, or a combination) to work on the reasons you think you can't say no or have to help everyone, even at your own expense.

* Use The Sweep to work with nonbeneficial beliefs (ideas) about boundaries (examples: *I have to help others* or *I'm mean, I'm not allowed to have boundaries, I'll never be able to feel okay unless I say yes to people*).

Commit to Yourself (Chapter 9)

Here I'm going to give you more ideas on how to honor those three commitments we learned about: telling yourself the truth, lightening up, and deciding to decide.

Tell Yourself the Truth

Telling yourself the truth is one of the hardest things to do. But it's also a necessary part of finding joy. Here are a few ways energy work can help you honor this commitment:

* Use The Sweep to clear the belief *Other people have to like my truth in order for me to be safe* or *My truth doesn't matter*.

* Use tapping (ATT, EFT, CT, or a combination) to tap and talk about all the reasons you are afraid to simply "know what you know" or clear unprocessed experiences where knowing or living your truth went bad in the past.

* Use TTT to release emotions making it hard for you to get in touch with your truth.

Lighten the F Up

As you know, beating up on yourself simply doesn't work to create a joyful life. Here are some ways to help you work toward lightening up on yourself:

* Use tapping (ATT, EFT, CT, or a combination) to clear unprocessed experiences linked to times when something bad happened because you made a mistake, times someone punished you for not doing something their way, and times where you feel you were judged or rejected for expressing yourself.

* Use The Sweep to clear the belief *I need to punish myself unless I do everything right*.

* Use TTT to release emotions contributing to self-criticism or to help support self-compassion.

Take Action/Decide

Not deciding your own life keeps you suspended in ambiguity and can feel like a constant panic attack or energy drain. Let's look at ways to get to quicker, easier decisions.

* Use The Sweep to clear the belief *There is only one right decision* or *I have to be 100 percent sure before I decide*.

* Use tapping (ATT, EFT, CT, or a combination) to work through feelings of fear about deciding.

* Use TTT to clear emotions blocking your clarity.

* Use tapping to release times from the past (unprocessed experiences) where you regret your decisions.

Muscle Testing (Chapter 10)

If you've had trouble with muscle testing, here are some ways to help you overcome it:

* Use TTT to release emotions interfering with easy and accurate muscle testing.

* Use tapping (ATT, EFT, CT, or a combination) to tap about the difficulties you're having with muscle testing.

* Use The Sweep to clear energy of pressure and stress around muscle testing.

* Use The Sweep to clear the belief *I need to be worried or fearful about the answers I get*.

Guide by Technique (Chapter 3)

Thymus Test and Tap (TTT)

You can use TTT to release emotions in so many different areas of life. Remember, there may be lots and lots of emotions stuck in your body. Each person can have thousands, but you don't need to clear even close to all of them in order to see improvement. TTT can produce pretty dramatic results, but you also know that working with it is a marathon and not a sprint. Make sure you're checking back several times to see if any new emotions are ready to come up and be released in relationship to any challenge you're working on.

Ask via muscle testing, *Can I find and release an emotion that is . . .*

* *disconnecting me from myself and life?*

* *contributing to depression/feeling bad/stress?*

* *making it difficult for me to heal from depression/feeling bad/stress?*

* *interfering with healthy chemical and hormonal balance in my body?*

* *related to a specific age in my life?* (If you get a "yes," you will need to muscle test to identify the age or choose an age.)

* *related to a specific experience from my past?* (If you get a "yes," you will need to muscle test to identify the age and figure out what happened at that time.)

* *triggered by a specific person in my life?* (If you get a "yes," you will need to muscle test to identify the person or choose a person to clear energy around. Remember that this is not a reason to blame anyone—it could even be linked to energy before you met them but they are just reminding you of it.)

* *linked to a specific place?* (If you get a "yes," you will
  need to muscle test to identify the place or choose a place
  to work with—for example, it could be a childhood home, a
  place of employment, a specific geographical location, etc.)

* *linked to a specific body part?* (Pay close attention to any parts of
  your body where there are physical symptoms.)

Tapping

Tapping, no matter which technique you're using (ATT, EFT, CT,
or a combination), is a great way to release stuck energy in your
body. Here are some effective ways you can use tapping:

* For any difficult feelings or situations or as a way to release
  stress, tension, and anxiety as it comes up

* To work with how you feel about dealing with depression
  (e.g., annoyed, frustrated, hopeless, etc.)

* To release unprocessed experiences from your past

* To clear beliefs (as an alternative or in addition to using
  The Sweep); for this, you'll simply use the tapping process
  and talk about the belief as you tap

The Sweep

The Sweep is a gentle yet powerful technique that helps you befriend
your subconscious mind to let go of old energy. With this technique,
you gently release energy that no longer serves you and install something positive. You learned how to use it for beliefs, but you can use it
to release any type of energy. Simply fill in the blank at the beginning
of the script with anything you want to release, such as the following:

* A belief

* A fear you have

* Energy related to a specific person, place, or thing (e.g., *career*, *my boss*, *enclosed spaces*, *my first boyfriend*, etc.)

* The phrase *all causes and contributing energy to* _____ (*depression*, *feeling bad*, etc.)

* Difficult feelings about a specific situation (e.g., *this frustration with not being able to get out of bed*)

* A physical symptom of depression (e.g., *fatigue*)

Build Your Own Sessions

Using all the different ideas I've provided you with can help you build your own energy sessions to work within. Simply mix and match whatever feels good and start releasing and clearing.

These sample sessions are ones I built quickly, pulling different parts of my approach and blending them for you just so you could see how your sessions could look—and how they're all perfectly right! Feel free to revise any of these session samples to meet your needs.

Sample Session #1

* Release five emotions from the past using TTT.

* Clear a belief from chapter 4 using The Sweep (three times in a row).

* Do an extra session of Tap + Breathe + Trace for five minutes.

Sample Session #2

* Use TTT to identify and clear emotions causing depression.

* Use TTT to identify and clear an area of the body with physical symptoms.

* Use tapping (ATT, EFT, CT, or a combination) to release feelings of doubt about the healing process.

* Use The Sweep to clear the belief *I'm unable to heal.*

Sample Session #3

* Use tapping (ATT, EFT, CT, or a combination) to work with calming the *freakout* response (see tapping script in appendix).

* Use TTT to identify and release emotions triggering panic in your body.

* Use The Sweep to clear *energy keeping me stuck.*

It is my great hope that you now have so many ideas for your healing that you'll refer back to them over and over again. These are the exact approaches that myself and thousands of others have used for their healing. Most important to remember, the problem all along has been all that you've been buried *under*. But *you* are just fine.

I know this life isn't always easy, and especially so with depression. I also know there are better days waiting for you. And as we remind each other in our house when someone is frustrated by the journey ahead, you're closer than you've ever been. And in fact, you're usually even closer than it feels.

May it be so for you too. Until then, I've got your back.

Acknowledgments

To Charlotte Phillips, my wife: I am eternally thankful for our *just-you-and-I-ness*. It never ever gets old. To my dearest friends and family, and especially to my mom (Ellen Scher): you are everything. It often takes a whole village to hold up just one author, and I couldn't feel more lucky to have you as part of mine.

To Steven Harris, my literary agent and forever friend, a million thank-yous are not enough. To the entire team at Sounds True, thank you. Tami Simon, a longtime inspiration of mine; Diana Ventimiglia, my fabulous editor and favorite Golden Girl; Leslie Brown, who made everything flow seamlessly; and Michelle Starika Asakawa, for her astute edits and attention to every word.

I cannot go without expressing my gratitude for all the people who support my work. An enormous thanks to my readers, who have taken the time to connect with me, both online and IRL. And to all the people out there who show up, often without recognition, to do such hard work for their healing . . . I'm proud of you.

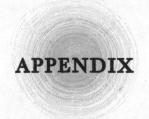

APPENDIX

Tapping Scripts

Here are a few tapping scripts to give you guidance on how to handle different challenges. I want you to use these scripts as templates to make your own for specific issues you are working on. Simply change the words to be relevant to your individual situation.

Subconscious Tapping Script #1

Use when you feel bad but aren't sure what's bothering you.

This script is for when you aren't sure exactly what to tap about or where to start. Here, we're going to utilize information in the subconscious mind, which already knows what's going on even if we can't quite figure it out. I call this "subconscious tapping" and I use it all the time.

Step 1: Start tapping on the karate-chop point continuously while repeating these statements:

Even though I feel so bad, I choose to let it go.

Even though I just feel bad, I choose to let it go.

Even though I feel so bad and don't know what's going on, I can be okay anyway.

Step 2: Cycle through the rest of the points using these statements as a guide (add your own or revise mine to feel more natural):

I feel so bad.

I hate feeling this way.

I feel it in my _____ (name part of body if you feel the emotion somewhere).

I don't know what to do, but my subconscious does.

I'm not sure why I am feeling like this.

My subconscious knows exactly what's going on.

My body remembers the details.

I just keep feeling _____.

I feel miserable.

This feeling is so _____ (describe it in detail—*scary, annoying, etc.*)

I am really struggling.

I'm not sure what it's from, but my subconscious does.

What we are doing in this part of the script is talking about or guessing about the details of why we feel like we do (even though it doesn't really matter). By "suggesting" ideas, the subconscious mind works behind the scenes to find those energies and clear them.

Step 3: Continue tapping for several more rounds, tapping through all the points while "venting" about how you feel, how you don't know why you feel this way, that your subconscious does, and so on.

Step 4: Wrap up with positive statements. Once you are happy with the improvement or need to finish your tapping session, do one more round using all positive statements.

I'm releasing old energy now.

I can be okay.

I am safe.

Subconscious Tapping Script #2

Use when you are working with vague memories or unprocessed experiences, including inherited, in utero, and past life.

Step 1: Start tapping on the karate-chop point continuously while repeating these statements:

Even though I have this experience _____ (fill in with the information you do know here—e.g., *something happened at age twenty with mom and I don't remember what it was*), *I give my subconscious permission to clear it anyway.*

Note: If it's a past-life or generational or other type of energy, you can just call it out as you tap by saying, *Even though I have this generational energy* _____ (and then fill in the details that you have).

Step 2: Cycle through the rest of the points using these statements as a guide (adding details of your experience in if you know them):

My subconscious knows exactly how to handle this old energy.

This event that happened _____ (state when it occurred including in a previous life, in utero, from your ancestors).

The details from that experience are _____ (all the smells, sights, and sounds; all the subconscious triggers).

I know it had something to do with _____.

My body knows the details.

I know that _____ (state what you do know/remember).

Step 3: Continue tapping for several more rounds, tapping through all the points while "venting" about the details you know.

Step 4: Wrap up with positive statements. Once you are happy with the improvement or need to finish your tapping session, do one more round using all positive statements.

I'm releasing old energy now.

I can move on now.

I am safe.

Calm the Nervous System Tapping Script

Use when you feel like you need to help shift your *freakout* response.

Step 1: Start tapping on the karate-chop point while repeating these statements:

Even though I feel freaked out (you can insert any other feelings you have here), *I choose to let it go.*

Even though I feel bad and stuck (you can insert any other feelings you have here), *I can be okay anyway.*

Even though I can't seem to get out of this, I can be okay anyway.

Step 2: Cycle through the rest of the points using these statements as a guide. Just "vent" about how you feel here. Anything you feel goes!

I just feel so _____ (describe how you feel here, using as many details as you'd like).

I feel ____ (shaky, nervous, sad, etc.).

I feel it in my _____ (name part of body, if you feel it anywhere in particular).

I'm not sure why I'm so stuck (if you have ideas, say, *I think* _____ *is what triggered me*).

My body is overwhelmed.

I just feel so stuck and don't even know what to do.

I want so badly to feel better.

But I feel _____.

All these frustrating feelings . . .

I feel so on edge.

All of this stuck energy in my body . . .

My body is in freakout *mode.*

It's hard to feel better.

Step 3: Continue tapping for several more rounds. Take a deep breath or two between every few rounds.

Step 4: Wrap up with positive statements. Once you are happy with the improvement or are done with your tapping session, do one more round using all positive statements. You can choose any of the following:

My system can calm down now.

I can be okay now.

I am safe.

Energetic Reactions Tapping Script

Use when you want to clear energy around things in your environment that you're reacting to.

Step 1: Start tapping on the karate-chop point while repeating these statements (adjust to what fits for you):

Even though I have this reaction to _____, I choose to let it go.

Even though my body can't yet handle _____, I can be okay anyway.

Even though my body doesn't seem to like _____, it's safe to release that reactive energy pattern.

Step 2: Cycle through the rest of the points using these statements as a guide:

My body doesn't like _____.

My body is really scared of _____.

For some reason my body doesn't like _____.

This strong reaction to _____.

My body got the idea that this _____ is scary!

This _____ is dangerous for me.

My body can't handle _____.

This strong reaction to _____.

My body doesn't like _____.

My body is really scared of _____.

For some reason my body doesn't like _____.

I'm so reactive to _____.

My body can't seem to handle _____.

Step 3: Continue tapping for several more rounds. Take a deep breath or two between every few rounds.

Step 4: Wrap up with positive statements. Once you are happy with the improvement or are done with your tapping session, do one more round using all positive statements. You can choose any of the following:

I'm ready to be friends with _____ now.

I can be perfectly okay with _____.

My body can relax around _____ now.

I'm willing to create a new pattern now. All can be well now.

I can easily handle _____ now. I'm okay.

I can feel at ease with _____.

It's time to relax. I can be okay.

_____ and I can coexist now.

I'm safe around _____ now. I'm okay.

In addition, the next time you do come in contact with the source of the reactive energy, I suggest that you use your tapping points to tap for about one minute before and after contact. You don't need to say anything, but rather just tap the points while in the presence of that energy in order to help reinforce the calm and balanced state. This typically needs to be done only with the first few contacts after clearing.

Note: Again, as a reminder, this practice is to use with negative energetic reactions. While people report being able to safely be in contact with things they couldn't before, allergies are a medical condition and you cannot rely on this practice for your health or safety.

Nightmares Tapping Script

Use when you can't sleep because of nightmares.

Remember that nightmares can be our mind's "playing out" worst-case scenarios to keep us safe. This is how we approach the issue using this tapping script.

Step 1: Start tapping on the karate-chop point continuously while repeating these statements:

Even though I just don't feel prepared to keep myself safe so I have to practice in the night, I can let this go.

Even though I have to practice saving my life or keeping myself safe while I sleep, I can change this.

Even though I need these nightmares to help me prepare for worst-case scenarios, I can let this pattern go.

Step 2: Cycle through the rest of the points using these statements as a guide:

I just can't trust that I'm safe.

I need to practice saving myself.

What if I don't know what to do and something bad happens?

I need to use my sleep time to train for worst-case scenarios.

I feel so unsafe all the time but even more so at night.

My subconscious knows how to help me let this go.

But I'm afraid to stop practicing.

I'm worried that I can't keep myself safe.

I need to "prepare" while I sleep.

These nightmares about _____ are keeping me safe.

I can't relax at night.

Something bad might happen and then I won't be ready.

Step 3: Continue tapping for several more rounds, tapping through all the points while "venting" about the nightmares and how you might be using them to keep you safe. Take a deep breath or two between every few rounds.

Step 4: Wrap up with positive statements. Once you are happy with the improvement or need to finish your tapping session, do one more round using all positive statements.

I can rest easily now.

I can be okay.

I am safe.

Energetic Sensitivity Tapping Script

Step 1: Start tapping on the karate-chop point continuously while repeating these statements:

Even though part of me is confused about what's mine and what's not, I choose to change this pattern.

Even though I have this pattern of taking on everyone else's stuff, I choose to let it go now.

Even though I am so sensitive to other people's energy, I give my body permission to let that go now.

Step 2: Cycle through the rest of the points using these statements as a guide:

I just feel things so intensely.

I seem to take things on without being aware.

Being around people feels so overwhelming to me.

I just pick up on everything around me.

I don't know how to stop it.

It makes me feel bad.

My body seems to do it automatically.

It's hard to hold my own boundaries.

This old pattern of taking on other people's stuff.

Continue tapping for several more rounds. Take a deep breath between rounds. Remember you are "venting" about how you feel and how this pattern affects you. That means any phrases that feel true for you will work.

Step 3: Wrap up with positive statements. Once you are happy with the improvement or are done with your tapping session, do one more round using all positive statements:

I can transform this old pattern.

I can have strong energetic boundaries.

I am safe.

Notes

Chapter 1—Why We Really Feel Like Shit (Even When There's "No Good Reason")

1. Candace B. Pert, *Molecules of Emotion: Why You Feel the Way You Feel* (New York: Scribner, 1997), 273.
2. Madhukar H. Trivedi, MD, "The Link Between Depression and Physical Symptoms," *Primary Care Companion to the Journal of Clinical Psychiatry* 6 (supplement 1), 2004: 12–16, ncbi.nlm.nih.gov/pmc/articles/PMC486942/.

Chapter 7—Listen to Your Body

1. Trivedi, "The Link Between Depression and Physical Symptoms," 12–16.

Chapter 9—Commit to Yourself: The Three Promises

1. Quoted in Olivia Campbell, "Keeping Secrets Isn't So Bad for You After All, with One Exception," *The Cut*, May 3, 2017, thecut.com/2017/05/keeping-secrets-isnt-bad-for-you-with-one-exception.html.
2. Emma Seppala, "The Scientific Benefits of Self-Compassion," Stanford University Center for Compassion and Altruism Research and Education, May 8, 2014, ccare.stanford.edu/uncategorized/the-scientific-benefits-of-self-compassion-infographic/.

3. Angus MacBeth and Andrew Gumley, "Exploring Compassion: A Meta-Analysis of the Association Between Self-Compassion and Psychopathology," National Institutes of Health, National Library of Medicine website, pubmed.ncbi.nlm.nih.gov/22796446/.

4. Sidney J. Blatt, "The Destructiveness of Perfectionism: Implications for the Treatment of Depression," *American Psychologist, 50*(12), 1995, 1003–1020. doi.org/10.1037/0003-066X.50.12.1003.

About the Author

AMY B. SCHER writes, teaches, and speaks on the topics "human-ing" and healing. As an energy therapist, she helps people release emotional baggage to become the happiest, healthiest version of themselves. She is the author of four books, which have been translated into thirteen languages and endorsed by notable authors such as Elizabeth Gilbert (*Eat, Pray, Love*), Vikas Swarup (*Slumdog Millionaire*), Bernie Siegel, MD (*Love, Medicine, and Miracles*), and Sanjiv Chopra, MD, MACP (*Brotherhood* with Deepak Chopra). Her work has appeared on CNN and CBS and in the *Washington Post, Cosmopolitan,* The Rumpus, *Los Angeles Review of Books,* and elsewhere. She lives in New York City with her beautiful wife and bad cat. Most importantly, she lives by her self-created motto: When life kicks your ass, kick back. She can be found online at AmyBScher.com.

About Sounds True

Sounds True is a multimedia publisher whose mission is to inspire and support personal transformation and spiritual awakening. Founded in 1985 and located in Boulder, Colorado, we work with many of the leading spiritual teachers, thinkers, healers, and visionary artists of our time. We strive with every title to preserve the essential "living wisdom" of the author or artist. It is our goal to create products that not only provide information to a reader or listener but also embody the quality of a wisdom transmission.

For those seeking genuine transformation, Sounds True is your trusted partner. At SoundsTrue.com you will find a wealth of free resources to support your journey, including exclusive weekly audio interviews, free downloads, interactive learning tools, and other special savings on all our titles.

To learn more, please visit SoundsTrue.com/freegifts or call us toll-free at 800.333.9185.

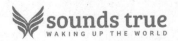